SURGERY – PROCEDURES, COMPLICATIONS, AND RESULTS

PROPHYLAXIS OF SURGICAL SITE INFECTION IN ABDOMINAL SURGERY

SURGERY – PROCEDURES, COMPLICATIONS, AND RESULTS

Additional books and e-books in this series can be found on Nova's website under the Series tab.

SURGERY – PROCEDURES, COMPLICATIONS, AND RESULTS

PROPHYLAXIS OF SURGICAL SITE INFECTION IN ABDOMINAL SURGERY

JAIME RUIZ-TOVAR, MD, PHD
AND
ANDRÉS GARCÍA MARÍN, MD, PHD
EDITORS

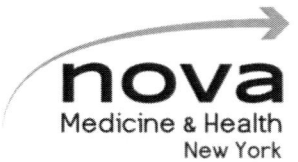

Copyright © 2019 by Nova Science Publishers, Inc.

All rights reserved. No part of this book may be reproduced, stored in a retrieval system or transmitted in any form or by any means: electronic, electrostatic, magnetic, tape, mechanical photocopying, recording or otherwise without the written permission of the Publisher.

We have partnered with Copyright Clearance Center to make it easy for you to obtain permissions to reuse content from this publication. Simply navigate to this publication's page on Nova's website and locate the "Get Permission" button below the title description. This button is linked directly to the title's permission page on copyright.com. Alternatively, you can visit copyright.com and search by title, ISBN, or ISSN.

For further questions about using the service on copyright.com, please contact:
Copyright Clearance Center
Phone: +1-(978) 750-8400   Fax: +1-(978) 750-4470   E-mail: info@copyright.com.

NOTICE TO THE READER

The Publisher has taken reasonable care in the preparation of this book, but makes no expressed or implied warranty of any kind and assumes no responsibility for any errors or omissions. No liability is assumed for incidental or consequential damages in connection with or arising out of information contained in this book. The Publisher shall not be liable for any special, consequential, or exemplary damages resulting, in whole or in part, from the readers' use of, or reliance upon, this material. Any parts of this book based on government reports are so indicated and copyright is claimed for those parts to the extent applicable to compilations of such works.

Independent verification should be sought for any data, advice or recommendations contained in this book. In addition, no responsibility is assumed by the Publisher for any injury and/or damage to persons or property arising from any methods, products, instructions, ideas or otherwise contained in this publication.

This publication is designed to provide accurate and authoritative information with regard to the subject matter covered herein. It is sold with the clear understanding that the Publisher is not engaged in rendering legal or any other professional services. If legal or any other expert assistance is required, the services of a competent person should be sought. FROM A DECLARATION OF PARTICIPANTS JOINTLY ADOPTED BY A COMMITTEE OF THE AMERICAN BAR ASSOCIATION AND A COMMITTEE OF PUBLISHERS.

Additional color graphics may be available in the e-book version of this book.

Library of Congress Cataloging-in-Publication Data

ISBN: 978-1-53615-615-7

Published by Nova Science Publishers, Inc. † New York

CONTENTS

Preface		**vii**
Chapter 1	Epidemiology of Surgical Site Infection *Pablo Priego*	1
Chapter 2	Adequate Nutritional Support for the Prophylaxis of Surgical Site Infection *Andrei Sarmiento, Grace Amesquita and Ramiro Carbajal*	19
Chapter 3	Preoperative Bath and Shave *Cristina Bernabeu Herraiz and Lorena Rodríguez Cazalla*	35
Chapter 4	Mechanical Bowel Preparation *Andrés García Marín and Mercedes Pérez López*	41
Chapter 5	Antibiotic Prophylaxis *Noel Rojas-Bonet and Maria del Mar García-Navarro*	47
Chapter 6	Hands and Skin Preparation *Lorena Rodríguez Cazalla and Cristina Bernabeu Herraiz*	55

Contents

Chapter 7	Hyperoxygenation, Hypothermia Prevention, Normoglycemia and Normovolemia *Esther García Villabona and Carmen Vallejo Lantero*	65
Chapter 8	Adhesives and Wound Protectors *Dennis César Lévano-Linares and Patricia Sanchez-Salcedo*	81
Chapter 9	Wound Irrigation *Gilberto González Ramírez*	93
Chapter 10	Topical Intraperitoneal Irrigation *Jaime Ruiz-Tovar and Carolina Llavero*	119
Chapter 11	Prophylactic Vacuum Therapy *Montiel Jiménez-Fuertes*	129
Chapter 12	Antimicrobial Sutures *Jaime Ruiz-Tovar and Carolina Llavero*	141
Chapter 13	Wound Cover: Topical Antibiotics or Antiseptics *Helen Almeida Ponce and Pablo Royo Dachary*	153
Chapter 14	Bundles *Camilo J. Castellón Pavón, Sonia Morales Artero, Elena Larraz Mora, Jaime Ruiz-Tovar and Manuel Durán Poveda*	171
About the Editors		189
Index		191
Related Nova Publications		199

PREFACE

Surgical-site infection (SSI) is a frequent complication after surgery and can be consider in certain circumstances a life-threatening condition. Three conditioning factors determine the development of SSI: the pathogen, the patient and the surgeon. The spectrum of pathogens causing SSI has not changed in the last decades, despite the incidence of antibiotic resistances to them have exponentially increased. The patient is a low-modifiable factor, but it is important a nutritional and comorbidities optimization. The surgeon is the most determinant factor on the development of SSI. It is important that the surgical act is correctly performed, with a correct management of tissues, preventing from unnecessary prolongation of the operative time, avoiding bleeding with a correct hemostasis and performing tension-free anastomoses, among other factors.

The surgeon has availability of several pharmacologic and non-pharmacologic measures to reduce the risk of SSI. Many of them have proven their efficacy in reducing SSI. However, a single measure is not enough to avoid SSI. Thus, bundles of measures have been developed, combining some of them, based on a synergistic effect on the reduction of SSI.

Recently, diverse scientific societies have published recommendations about different measures to reduce SSI, indicating that this entity has become a priority in health care, as the sanitary costs derived from SSI overcome the investment on different devices, drugs or measures to prevent SSI.

We hope that this book, based on the current evidence on prophylactic measures to prevent SSI, can be helpful in the clinical practice. However, we must keep always in mine, that medical investigation obtains new data, drugs and approaches every day, so that current evidence can be outdated in the following decade, requiring future updates.

Finally, we want to thank to all the contributing authors, all of them friends and experts in their corresponding fields, their availability, time and efforts to write all the chapters.

Jaime Ruiz-Tovar, MD, PhD
Andrés Garcia-Marin, MD, PhD
Editors

In: Prophylaxis of Surgical Site Infection ...   ISBN: 978-1-53615-615-7
Editors: Jaime Ruiz-Tovar et al.   © 2019 Nova Science Publishers, Inc.

Chapter 1

EPIDEMIOLOGY OF SURGICAL SITE INFECTION

Pablo Priego[*], *MD, PhD*

Department of General Surgery, Division of Esophagogastric and Bariatric Surgery, Ramón y Cajal University Hospital, Madrid, Spain

ABSTRACT

Surgical site infection (SSI) refers to an infection that occurs within 30 days after surgery in the part of the body where the surgery took place. These infections may be superficial (involving the skin only) or deep incisional infections or infections involving organs, implanted materials or body spaces. True epidemiology of SSI is difficult to identify due to the heterogeneous nature of these infections. In fact, incidence can change between procedures, hospitals, surgeons and patients. SSIs are the first most frequently reported nosocomial infections, accounting for 30% of such infections among hospitalised patients. Moreover, SSI is implicated in one-third of postoperative deaths and accounts for 8% of all deaths caused by a nosocomial infection. Furthermore, SSI incurs considerable increases in healthcare costs. In most SSIs, the responsible pathogens originate from the patient's endogenous flora. The most

---

[*] Corresponding Author's Email: papriego@hotmail.com.

commonly isolated organisms in clean surgery are *Staphylococcus aureus*, coagulase negative staphylococci, meanwhile in clean-contaminated or contaminated surgery; the most frequent organisms are *Enterococcus* spp. and Escherichia *coli*.

This review aims at exploring epidemiology, bacteriology and risk factors associated with SSI.

Keywords: epidemiology, surgical site infection, microbiology, risk factors, pathogens

HISTORY

The introduction of anesthetics encouraged more surgery, which inadvertently caused more dangerous patient post-operative infections. The concept of infection was unknown until relatively modern times.

The modern concept of asepsis evolved in the 19th century, when Ignaz Semmelweis showed that hand washing prior to delivery reduced puerperal fever [1]. However, until the pioneering work of Joseph Lister in the 1860s, most physicians believed that chemical damage from exposures to bad air (miasma) was responsible for infections in wounds, and facilities for washing hands or a patient's wounds were not available.

Lister became aware of the work of chemist Louis Pasteur, who showed that rotting and fermentation could occur under anaerobic conditions if micro-organisms were present. Lister experienced spraying carbolic acid on his instruments as an antiseptic, and found that this remarkably reduced the incidence of gangrene and surgical site infections (SSIs). His work was groundbreaking and laid the foundations for a rapid advance in infection control that saw modern antiseptic operating theatres widely used within 50 years [1].

Nowadays, strategies for the prevention of SSIs are based both on reducing the risk of bacterial contamination and on improving the patient's defences against infection. This requires a 'bundle' approach, with attention to multiple patient-related and procedure-related risk factors. Evidence-based guidelines for the prevention of SSIs have been published by the Centers for Disease Control (CDC) [2] and World Health Organitation [3]. However, the development of such guidelines is complicated by the heterogeneous nature of SSIs, which makes it difficult to generalise findings from a study in a specific patient population to a wider setting, and by the fact that the impact of many routine practices (e.g., wearing surgical gloves) cannot be evaluated for ethical or logistic reasons.

DEFINITION

The expression 'surgical site infection' (SSI) was introduced in 1992 in order to replace the previous concept of 'surgical wound infection' [4]. SSI refers to an infection that occurs after surgery in the part of the body where the surgery took place. These infections may be superficial (involving the skin only) or deep incisional infections, or infections involving organs, implanted materials or body spaces (Figure 1).

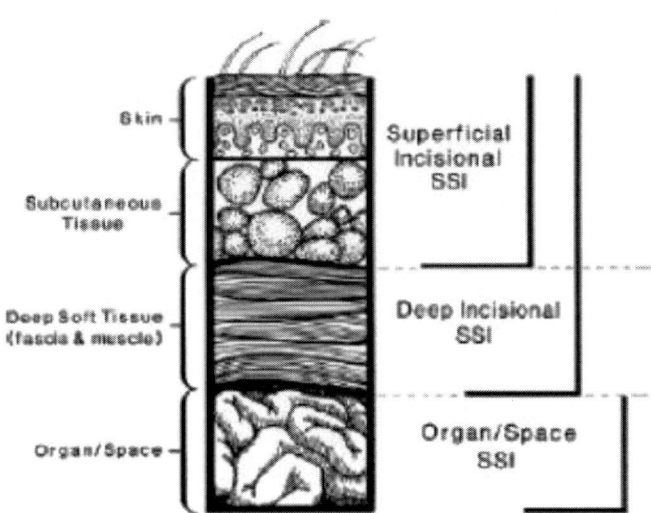

Figure 1. Classification of SSIs according to the Centers for Disease Control National Nosocomial Infections Surveillance (CDC NNIS) System. Reproduced with permission from Mangram et al. [5].

Criterion	CDC 1988	CDC 1992	SISG	NPS	PHLS
Purulent discharge in or exuding from the wound or observed on direct examination	I		✓	✓	✓
Painful spreading erythema indicative of cellulitis			✓	✓	
Purulent drainage	D	SI/D			
Purulent drainage from a drain placed beneath the fascial layer	D				
Purulent drainage from a drain placed through a stab wound into the organ/space		OS			
Organisms isolated from fluid or tissue from the wound	I	SI			
Organisms isolated from fluid or tissue in the organ/space		OS			
Surgeon/physician diagnosis	I/D	SI/DI/OS			
Surgeon deliberately opens wound, unless wound is culture-negative	I/D	SI/DI			
Wound spontaneously dehisces	D	SI/DI			
Pain	D	SI/DI			
Tenderness	D	DI	✓	✓	
Fever > 38°C	D	DI	✓	✓	
Localized swelling (oedema)		SI	✓	✓	
Redness or extending margin or erythema		SI	✓	✓	
Patient still receiving active treatment for a wound with discharged pus				or ✓	
Heat		SI			
Abscess or other evidence of infection found on direct examination	D	DI/OS			

*Reproduced from reference 4.
CDC: Centers for Disease Control and Prevention; SISG: Surgical Infection Study Group; NPS: National Prevalence Survey; PHLS: Public Health Laboratory Service.
CDC 1988 definitions: I, incisional surgical wound infection; D, deep surgical wound infection. CDC 1992 definitions: SI, superficial incisional; DI, deep incisional; OS, organ/space. The SISG and NPS allow fever (>38°C), tenderness, oedema, an extending margin of erythema or if the patient is still receiving treatment for the wound.

Figure 2. Definitions of SSI (Reproduced with permission from Global guidelines for the prevention of surgical site infection. World Health Organization (2016) [3].

SSI is also defined as an infection that occurs within 30 days after the operation and involves the skin and subcutaneous tissue of the incision (superficial incisional) and/or the deep soft tissue (for example, fascia, muscle) of the incision (deep incisional) and/or any part of the anatomy (for example, organs and spaces) other than the incision that was opened or manipulated during an operation (organ/space) [3].

There are many definitions of SSI and a systematic review identified as many as 41 different definitions. However, only five were described as being standardized definitions created by multidisciplinary groups (Figure 2).

The period of surveillance during the first 30 postoperative days or 1 year in case of receiving implants has been modified in the last years by CDC. Currently, it has been stablished two different kind of clasiffications regarding procedures and these period of surveillance change from 30 to 90 days in them (Table 1) [6].

Table 1. Period of surveillance for deep or organ/space surgical infection recommended by CDC (2015)

Period of surveillance for deep or organ/space surgical infection recommended by CDC (2015)	
Surveillance of 30 days	Surveillance of 90 days
Aortic aneurysm	Breast surgery
Amputation of extremity	Herniorraphy
Appendectomy	Implanting a pacemaker
Hepatobiliopancreatic surgery	Peripheral vascular surgery
Cholecystectomy	Hip and knee prosthesis
Colorectal surgery	Spinal surgery
Gastric surgery	Craneothomy
Small bowel surgery	Open bone fracture
Neck, thyroid an parathyroid surgery	
Splenectomy	
Explorer laparoscopy	
Ovarian surgery	
Abdominal or vaginal hysterectomy	
Caesarean surgery	
Kidney, liver and cardiac transplantation	
Thoracic surgery	
Superficial SSIs are only controlled for 30 days with independence of type of surgery	

Surgical Wound [3]

Surgical wound refers to a wound created when an incision is made with a scalpel or other sharp cutting device and then closed in the operating room by suture, staple, adhesive tape, or glue and resulting in close approximation to the skin edges.

Surgical wounds are classified according to level of contamination into four classes. This classification allow a better prediction of risk of infections and wound healing outcomes, thus allowing most favorable treatment for each type of surgical wound.

Clean: refers to an uninfected operative wound in which no inflammation is encountered and the respiratory, alimentary, genital or uninfected urinary tracts are not entered. In addition, clean wounds are primarily closed and, if necessary, drained with closed drainage. Operative incisional wounds that follow non-penetrating (blunt) trauma should be included in this category if they meet the criteria.

Clean-contaminated: refers to operative wounds in which the respiratory, alimentary, genital or urinary tracts are entered under controlled conditions and without unusual contamination. Specifically, operations involving the biliary tract, appendix, vagina and oropharynx are included in this category, provided no evidence of infection or major break in technique is encountered.

Contaminated: refers to open, fresh, accidental wounds. In addition, operations with major breaks in sterile technique (for example, open cardiac massage) or gross spillage from the gastrointestinal tract, and incisions in which acute, non-purulent inflammation is encountered, including necrotic tissue without evidence of purulent drainage (for example, dry gangrene), are included in this category.

Dirty or infected: includes old traumatic wounds with retained devitalized tissue and those that involve existing clinical infection or perforated viscera. This definition suggests that the organisms causing postoperative infection were present in the operative field before the operation.

EPIDEMIOLOGY

SSIs are a common cause of healthcare-associated infection (HAI). True epidemiology of SSI is difficult to identify due to the heterogeneous nature of these infections. In fact, incidence can change between procedures, hospitals, surgeons and patients [7]. Data from the United States and Spain show that SSIs are the first most frequently reported nosocomial infections, accounting for 30% of such infections among hospitalised patients. Furthermore, SSI is a serious complication of surgical procedures that occurs after approximately 2-7% of surgeries. However, its incidence depends on the surgical procedure, the surveillance criteria used, and the quality of data collection.

Moreover, SSI is the most common complication following major gastrointestinal surgery, affecting between 25% and 40% of patients after midline laparotomy (especially in transplantation and surgical oncology) [8]. Fortunately, the increasing use of minimally invasive surgery approach has resulted in a decrease in the incidence of SSIs.

Actually, SSI occurs 17 days after surgery with a range of 6-41 days. In colorectal surgery, 70% of SSI develops after discharge home [9].

Impact of SSIs on Healthcare Resources

SSI is implicated in one-third of postoperative deaths and accounts for 8% of all deaths caused by a nosocomial infection. Furthermore, SSIs cause pain and discomfort, increase hospital stay, require readmission to hospital or intensive care unit (ICU) treatment, and deffinitively put patients at greater risk of secondary infectious complications [5].

Kirkland et al. [10], reported that the relative risk for death associated with SSIs was 2.2, and those for readmission and ICU treatment were 5.5 and 1.6, respectively. Moreover, patients with SSIs required longer hospitalization (11 vs. 6 days) when compared with uninfected patients, and the median extra duration attributable to SSIs was between 5 to 10 days [11].

As a result, SSIs incur considerable increases in healthcare costs. The hospital-related cost of a single SSI has been estimated at $12,000–$35,000 and estimates of annual nationwide hospital costs of SSI have ranged from $3 billion to $10 billion [12].

MICROBIOLOGY

In most SSIs, the responsible pathogens originate from the patient's endogenous flora. Type of organisms isolated depends on type of surgery. The most commonly isolated organisms in clean surgery are *Staphylococcus aureus*, coagulase negative staphylococci, meanwhile in clean-contaminated or contaminated surgery, the most frequent organisms are *Enterococcus* spp. and *Escherichia coli* [13, 14].

Results form EPINE study of Spain in 2013 [15], shows that in gastrointestinal surgery, SSI is secondary to gram-negative germens in 60% and gram-positive cocos in 32%. Most frequent isolated organisms are *Escherichia coli* (28%), *Enterococcus* spp. (15%), *Streptococcus* spp. (8%), *Pseudomonas aeruginosa* (7%), coagulase negative staphylococci (5%), *Staphylococcus aureus* (5%, methicilin-resistant 2%), *Candida spp.* (4%), *Klebsiella* spp. (4%), *Enterobacter* spp. (4%), *Proteus mirabilis* (3%) and *Bacteroides fragilis* (3%) [6].

Nowadays, there are an increase proportion of infections caused by pathogens antimicrobial resistance, like methicilin-resistant *Staphylococcus aureus* (MRSA) or *Candida*. This could be indicative to the increasing number of immunocompromised surgical patients or even severely ill, as well as to the widespread overuse of broad-spectrum antibiotics. This MRSA infection not only is associated with long and expensive hospitalizations but also with high mortality rates.

Less frequent are infections caused by *Serratia marcescens, Moxarella osloensis, Rhizopus oryzae, Clostridium perfringens, Rhodococcus bronchialis, Nocardia farcinica, Legionella pneumophila, Legionella dumoffii* and *Pseudomonas multivorans*. However, when these infections are detected, a meticulous epidemiologic investigation must be taking.

Pathogens of concern that cause SSIs may be introduced to the site of wound or surgery via several routes like the patient's endogenous flora or preoperative infection sites remote from the operative, particularly in patients undergoing insertion of a prosthesis or other implant. In addition to the patient's endogenous flora, SSI pathogens may originate from exogenous sources such as members of the surgical team, the operating theatre environment, and instruments and materials brought within the sterile field during the procedure.

The risk of an SSI developing after microbial contamination of the surgical site will depend on the dose and virulence of the pathogen and the patient's level of resistance, according to the relationship

$$\text{Risk of SSI} = \frac{\text{Dose of bacterial contamination} \times \text{virulence}}{\text{Resistance of patient}}$$

The risk of SSI is considered to be significant when organisms in the tissue exceed 105 organisms per gram of tissue, although lower doses may be required if foreign material such as sutures is present. The virulence of the organism relates to its ability to produce toxins or other factors that increase its ability to invade or damage tissue. When the balance between the patient's defense system and the number of pathogenic organisms is disrupted SSIs occur. Mortality rates in patients infected with highly virulent pathogens such as MRSA may be as high as 74% [7].

RISKS FACTORS FOR SSIS

A number of patient-related and procedure-related factors have been shown to influence the risk of SSIs (Table 2). These include patient-related (endogenous factors) and procedure-related (exogenous factors). Some variables are obviously not modifiable, such as age and gender. However, other potential factors can be improved to increase the likelihood of a positive surgical outcome, such as nutritional status, tobacco use, correct use of antibiotics and the intraoperative technique [7].

The risk of SSI in an individual patient can be estimated using various scoring systems. Culver et al. in 1991 [16], reported the National Nosocomial Infections Surveillance (NNIS) SSI Risk Index. This is the most frequent index in order to calculate the probability of SSI. This index has a range of 0-3, and is calculated by assigning one point for each of three variables (Table 3):

a) Duration of surgery longer than the approximate 75th percentile of the duration of the specific operation being performed (1 point)
b) Type of surgery: The presence of a contaminated, dirty or infected, wound (1 point)
c) Classification of the American Society of Anesthesiologists score: A score of > 3 (i.e., mild systemic disease) is assigned with 1 point.

Table 2. Patient-related and procedure-related factors that may influence the risk of surgical site infections (adapted from Mangram et al.) [5]

Patient-related	Procedure-related
Age	Duration of surgical scrub
Nutritional status	Skin antisepsis
Diabetes	Preoperative shaving
Smoking	Preoperative skin preparation
Obesity	Duration of operation
Coexistent infection at a remote body site	Antimicrobial prophylaxis
Colonisation with micro-organisms	Operating room ventilation
(particularly *Staphylococcus aureus*)	Inadequate sterilisation of surgical instruments
Altered immune response	
Length of preoperative hospital stay	Foreign material in the surgical site
	Surgical drains
	Surgical technique
	-poor haemostasis
	-failure to obliterate dead space
	-tissue trauma

Korol et al. [17] performe a systematic review of 57 studies and identify an increased risk of SSI with the following factors: a high body mass index, a severe score according to the US National Nosocomial Infections Surveillance (NNIS) risk Index, severe wound class, diabetes and a prolongation of surgery duration. Furthermore, a metaanalysis of Zhang et al. [18], suggested that diabetes mellitus is significantly associated with an increased risk of SSI. Indeed, in European studies [19], it has also been identified a longer duration of surgery, an American

Society of Anesthesiologists score of at least 3 and a pre-surgery hospital stay of at least 2 days as factors associated with an increased risk of SSI, while videoscopic procedures reduced SSI rates.

Table 3. Estimation of preoperative SSI risk based on the National Nosocomial Infections Surveillance System (NNISS)

Estimation of preoperative SSI risk based on the National Nosocomial Infections Surveillance System (NNISS)		
NNISS		
1- Duration of surgery longer than the approximate 75th percentile of the duration of the specific operation being performed (1 point) 2-Type of surgery: The presence of a contaminated, dirty or infected, wound (1 point) 3- ASA score of ≥ 3 is assigned with 1 point.		
KEYS		
ASA I	A normal healthy patient	
ASA II	A patient with mild systemic disease	
ASA III	A patient with severe systemic disease	
ASA IV	A patient with severe systemic disease that is a constant threat to life	
ASA V	A moribund patient who is not expected to survive without the operation	
ASA VI	A declared brain-dead patient whose organs are being removed for donor purposes	
T: Cross point for surgery		
Appendectomy	1 hour	
Pancreas, liver and biliar tract surgery	4 hours	
Cholecystectomy	2 hours	
Colon surgery	3 hours	
Gastric surgery	3 hours	
Smallo bowel surgery	3 hours	
Laparotomy	2 hours	
Another procedures in the digestive tract	3 hours	
RISK OF INFECTION		
0 points: 1.5% 1 point: 2.9% 2 points: 6.8% 3 points: 13%		

Recently, a systematic review conducted by WHO [20-33], tried to describe the relationship between surgical volume and the risk of SSI. A moderate quality of evidence showed that surgical procedures performed in high-/medium volume hospitals have lower SSI rates compared to low-volume hospitals (OR: 0.69; 95% CI: 0.55-0.87 and OR: 0.80; 95% CI: 0.69-0.94, respectively). In addition, there was a moderate quality of evidence that surgical procedures performed by high- or medium-volume surgeons have lower SSI rates (OR: 0.67; 95% CI: 0.55-0.81 and OR: 0.73; 95% CI: 0.63-0.85, respectively) compared to low volume hospitals. However, there was controversial evidence when high- and medium-volume hospitals were compared and it remains unclear whether there is a linear relationship between procedure/surgeon volume and the SSI rate.

CLASSIFICATION OF THE SEVERITY OF THE SSI: THE ASEPSIS SCORE

Having a valid, reliable and sensitive scoring system to assess the signs and symptoms of SSI can allow prompt treatment as well as evaluation of its management. The ASEPSIS scoring system, derived from cardiac surgery, was the only established referenced scoring system to assess for SSI. The acronym of ASEPSIS is *Additional treatment, Serous discharge, Erythema, Purulent exudates, Separation of deep tissues, Isolation of bacteria and Stay as inpatient prolonged over fourteen days* [34].

ASEPSIS score evaluates the severity of SSI during the first postoperative week assigning points to several factors (antibiotics, drainage of pus, debridement, evisceration, microbiology). This score classifies postoperative infection in five categories (from satisfactory healing to severe infection) and may evaluate daily the score [6] (Table 4).

Table 4. ASEPSIS score

	Proportion of wound affected (%)					
Wound characteristics	0	< 20	20-39	40-50	60-79	>80
Serous exudates	0	1	2	3	4	5
Erythema	0	1	2	3	4	5
Purulent exudates	0	2	4	6	8	10
Separation of Deep tissues	0	2	4	6	8	10

Criteria	Points
Additional treatment	
-Antibiotics	10
-Drainage of pus under local anesthesia	5
-Debridement of wound general anesthesia	10
Serous discharge	Daily 0-5
Erythema	Daily 0-5
Purulent exudates	Daily 0-10
Separation of deep tissues	Daily 0-10
Isolation of bacteria	10
Stay as inpatient prolonged over 14 days	5
Total score	**Category of infection**
0-10	Satisfactory healing
11-20	Disturbance of healing
21-30	Minor wound infection
31-40	Moderate wound infection
>40	Severe wound infection

REFERENCES

[1] Thorwald J (2005). Das Jahrhundert der Chirurgen. [The Century of Surgeons.] *Edition Destino*, S.A. Pag 1-662.

[2] Berríos-Torres SI, Umscheid CA, Bratzler DW, Leas B, Stone EC, Kelz RR, Reinke CE, Morgan S, Solomkin JS, Mazuski JE, Dellinger EP, Itani KMF, Berbari EF, Segreti J, Parvizi J, Blanchard J, Allen G, Kluytmans JAJW, Donlan R, Schecter WP for the Healthcare Infection Control Practices Advisory Committee (2017). Centers for

Disease Control and Prevention Guideline for the Prevention of Surgical Site Infection, 2017. *JAMA Surg*;152(8):784-791.

[3] *Global guidelines for the prevention of surgical site infection.* World Health Organization (2016). Pag. 1-186.

[4] Horan TC, Gaynes RP, Martone WJ, Jarvis WR, Emori TG (1992). CDC definitions of noscomial surgical site infections, 1992: a modification of CDC definitions of surgical wound infections. *Infect Control Hosp Epidemiol*; 13: 606-608.

[5] Mangram AJ, Horan TC, Pearson ML, Silver LC, Jarvis WR (1999). Hospital Infection Control Practice Advisory Committee. Guideline for prevention of surgical site infection, 1999. *Infect Control Hosp Epidemiol*; 20: 247-278.

[6] Badía JM (2016). Surgical site infection: definition, classification and risk factors. *Clinical guidelines of Spanish Association of Surgeons. Surgical Infections.* Aran SL. 2ª edición. Pag. 97-116.

[7] Owens CD, Stoessel K (2008). Surgical site infections: epidemiology, microbiology and prevention. *Journal of Hospital Infection*; 70(S2) 3–10.

[8] Collaborative GS (2017). Determining the worldwide epidemiology of surgical site infections after gastrointestinal resection surgery: protocol for a multicentre, international, prospective cohort study (GlobalSurg 2). *BMJ Open*;7:e012150. doi:10.1136/ bmjopen-2016-012150.

[9] Limón E, Shaw E, Badia JM, Piriz M, Escofet R, Gudiol F, Pujol M (2014). Post-discharge surgical site infections after uncomplicated elective colorectal surgery: impact and risk factors. The experience of the VINCat Program. *J Hosp Infection*; 86:127-132.

[10] Kirkland KB, Briggs JP, Trivette SL, Wilkinson WE, Sexton DJ (1999). The impact of surgical-site infections in the 1990s: attributable mortality, excess length of hospitalization, and extra costs. *Infect Control Hosp Epidemiol*; 20:725-730.

[11] DiPiro JT, Martindale RG, Bakst A, Vacani PF, Watson P, Miller MT (1998). Infection in surgical patients: effects on mortality,

hospitalization, and postdischarge care. *Am J Health Syst Pharm*; 55:777-781.

[12] Baker AW, Dicks KV, Durkin MJ, Weber DJ, Lewis SS, Moehring RW, Chen LF, Sexton DJ, Anderson DJ (2016). Epidemiology of Surgical Site Infection in a Community Hospital Network. *Infect Control Hosp Epidemiol*; 37(5): 519–526.

[13] Múñez E, Ramos A, Álvarez de Espejo T, Vaque J, Sánchez-Payá J, Pastor V, Asensio A (2011).Microbiology of surgical site infections in abdominal tract surgery patients. *Cir Esp*; 89:606-612.

[14] Magill, SS, et al. (2012) Prevalence of healthcare-associated infections in acute care hospitals in Jacksonville, Florida. *Infection Control Hospital Epidemiology*; 33(3):283-291.

[15] Estudio EPINE-EPPS 2013. *Study of prevalence of nosocomial infections in Spain.*

[16] Culver DH, Horan TC, Gaynes RP, Martone WJ, Jarvis WR, Emori TG, Banerjee SN, Edwards JR, Tolson JS, Henderson TS, Hughes JM, and the National Nosocomial Infections Surveillance System (1991). Surgical wound infection rates by wound class, operative procedure, and patient risk index. *Am J Med*; 91:152S-157S.

[17] Korol E, Johnston K, Waser N, Sifakis F, Jafri HS, Lo M, et al. (2013). A systematic review of risk factors associated with surgical site infections among surgical patients. *PLoS One*; 8(12):e83743.

[18] Zhang Y, Zheng QJ, Wang S, Zeng SX, Zhang YP, Bai XJ, et al. (2015). Diabetes mellitus is associated with increased risk of surgical site infections: A meta-analysis of prospective cohort studies. *Am J Infect Control;*43(8):810-815.

[19] Marchi M, Pan A, Gagliotti C, Morsillo F, Parenti M, Resi D, et al. (2014). The Italian national surgical site infection surveillance programme and its positive impact, 2009 to 2011. *Euro Surveill*;19(21): pii: 20815.

[20] Anderson DJ, Hartwig MG, Pappas T, Sexton DJ, Kanafani ZA, Auten G, et al. (2008). Surgical volume and the risk of surgical site infection in community hospitals: size matters. *Ann Surg*; 247(2):343-349.

[21] Hervey SL, Purves HR, Guller U, Toth AP, Vail TP, Pietrobon R (2003). Provider volume of total knee arthroplasties and patient outcomes in the HCUP nationwide inpatient sample. *J Bone Joint Surg (Am)*;85-a(9):1775-1783.

[22] Jalisi S, Bearelly S, Abdillahi A, Truong MT (2013). Outcomes in head and neck oncologic surgery at academic medical centers in the United States. *Laryngoscope*; 123(3):689-698.

[23] Meyer E, Weitzel-Kage D, Sohr D, Gastmeier P (2011). Impact of department volume on surgical site infections following arthroscopy, knee replacement or hip replacement. *BMJ Qual Saf*; 20(12):1069-1074.

[24] Muilwijk J, van den Hof S, Wille JC (2007). Associations between surgical site infection risk and hospital operation volume and surgeon operation volume among hospitals in the Dutch nosocomial infection surveillance network. *Infect Control Hosp Epidemiol*; 28(5):557-563.

[25] Namba RS, Inacio MC, Paxton EW (2012). Risk factors associated with surgical site infection in 30,491 primary total hip replacements. *J Bone Joint Surg (Br)*; 94(10):1330-1338.

[26] Patel HJ, Herbert MA, Drake DH, Hanson EC, Theurer PF, Bell GF, et al. (2013). Aortic valve replacement: using a statewide cardiac surgical database identifies a procedural volume hinge point. *Ann Thorac Surg*; 96(5):1560-1565; discussion 5-6.

[27] Wu SC, Chen CC, Ng YY, Chu HF (2006). The relationship between surgical site infection and volume of coronary artery bypass graft surgeries: Taiwan experience. *Infect Control Hosp Epidemiol*; 27(3):308-311.

[28] Geubbels EL, Wille JC, Nagelkerke NJ, Vandenbroucke-Grauls CM, Grobbee DE, de Boer AS (2005). Hospital-related determinants for surgical site infection following hip arthroplasty. *Infect Control Hosp Epidemiol*; 26(5):435-441.

[29] Katz JN, Losina E, Barrett J, Phillips CB, Mahomed NN, Lew RA, et al. (2001). Association between hospital and surgeon procedure volume and outcomes of total hip replacement in the United States medicare population. *J Bone Joint Surg (Am);* 83-a(11):1622-1629.

[30] Katz JN, Barrett J, Mahomed NN, Baron JA, Wright RJ, Losina E (2004). Association between hospital and surgeon procedure volume and the outcomes of total knee replacement. *J Bone Joint Surg (Am)*; 86-a(9):1909-1916.

[31] Kreder HJ, Deyo RA, Koepsell T, Swiontkowski MF, Kreuter W (1997). Relationship between the volume of total hip replacements performed by providers and the rates of postoperative complications in the state of Washington. *J Bone Joint Surg (Am)*; 79(4):485-494.

[32] Nguyen NT, Paya M, Stevens CM, Mavandadi S, Zainabadi K, Wilson SE (2004). The relationship between hospital volume and outcome in bariatric surgery at academic medical centers. *Ann Surg*; 240(4):586-593.

[33] Shah SN, Wainess RM, Karunakar MA (2005). Hemiarthroplasty for femoral neck fracture in the elderly surgeon and hospital volumerelated outcomes. *J Arthroplasty*; 20(4):503-508.

[34] Leaper DJ (2010). Risk factors for and Epidemiology of Surgical Site Infections. *Surg Infect;* 11(3): 283-287.

In: Prophylaxis of Surgical Site Infection ... ISBN: 978-1-53615-615-7
Editors: Jaime Ruiz-Tovar et al. © 2019 Nova Science Publishers, Inc.

Chapter 2

ADEQUATE NUTRITIONAL SUPPORT FOR THE PROPHYLAXIS OF SURGICAL SITE INFECTION

Andrei Sarmiento[1,*], *MD, Grace Amesquita*[2], *MD and Ramiro Carbajal*[3], *MD*

[1]Metabolic and Bariatric Surgeon, Hospital Santa Rosa, Lima, Perú
[2]Intensive care unit (ICU), Hospital Santa Rosa, Lima, Perú
[3]Metabolic and Bariatric Surgeon,
Hospital Edgardo Rebagliati, Lima, Perú

ABSTRACT

Surgical site infections (SSI) are one of the most commonly reported healthcare-associated infections worldwide and have adverse effects on patient health and hospital resources. There are several risk factors to develop SSI and include malnutrition. A large part of all patients in the hospital are at nutritional risk, the prevalence of malnutrition is up to 50-55%. Due to this high prevalence current recommendations to avoid the hospital burden to SSIs include identify the presence of malnutrition

---

[*] Corresponding Author's Email: andreisarmiento@hotmail.com.

adopting specific nutritional goals to preoperative and postoperative period.

Keywords: surgical site infections, malnutrition, nutritional support

INTRODUCTION

According to the World Health Organization (WHO) healthcare-associated infections are avoidable infections that affect hundreds of millions of people each year worldwide, and surgical site infection (SSI) is the most frequent healthcare-associated infection in low-income countries, affecting up to a third of patients who had surgery. The incidence of SSI is much lower in high-income countries, while urinary tract infection is the most frequent. SSI is still the second most common in Europe and the USA. In low and middle-income countries the incidence rates ranging from 1.2 to 23.6 per 100 surgical procedures and a pooled incidence of 11.8%. By contrast, SSI rates vary between 1.2% and 5.2% in developed countries [1, 2].

Surgical site infection (SSI) is defined by the United States Centers for Disease Control and Prevention as infection related to an operative procedure that occurs at or near the surgical incision within 30 days of the procedure or within 90 days if prosthetic material is implanted at surgery [3].

Several risk factors predispose SSI and are known in the literature. Patient and operation characteristics that may influence the risk of surgical site infection development according to the Centers for Disease Control and Prevention guideline. Patient factors include (age, nutritional status, diabetes, smoking, obesity, coexistent infections at a remote body site, colonization with microorganisms, altered immune response length of preoperative stay). Procedure factors include the duration of surgical scrub, skin antisepsis, preoperative shaving, preoperative skin preparation, duration of operation, antimicrobial prophylaxis, operating room ventilation, inadequate sterilization of instruments, foreign material in the surgical site, surgical techniques, surgical drains) [3, 4]. There are other factors influencing patient to develop SSI for example, Hypoalbuminemia [5].

Nowadays, the relationship between nutritional status and the immune system is well known. Malnutrition impairs immune response may make patients highly susceptible to postoperative infections. Hence, patients with malnutrition may suffer a range of poor outcomes including increased risk of death, sepsis and poor wound healing [6, 7]. This chapter summarizes the recent evidence about the identification and intervention of the malnutrition in the surgical patient to avoid surgical site infections.

MALNUTRITION AS A RISK FACTOR

About 20%–50% of all patients in hospitals are found at risk of undernutrition, depending on the definition, clinical setting, and screening tools. A large part of these patients at nutritional risk when admitted to the hospital, and in most of the patient's malnutrition develops negatively during the hospital stay [6]. The elderly patients and patients suffering from chronic diseases are more exposed to nutritional risk than other patients [7, 8]. Despite three decades of collective development of knowledge, contemporary malnutrition rates do not appear to have reduced significantly [9]. This can be prevented if special attention is paid to the nutritional care of patients.

Malnutrition is characterized by the presence of two or more of the following characteristics: Insufficient energy intake, weight loss, loss of muscle mass, loss of subcutaneous fat, localized or generalized fluid accumulation or decreased functional status [10].

In general, contributors to adult malnutrition have been described in a number of recent studies. Factors identified include inadequate intake, inadequate access to food, increased nutrient requirements associated with complications of the presenting disease or condition, complications that develop during the course of a hospital stay, and/or complications that occur as a result of treatment, declines in mental, sensory, and/or physical function, changes in metabolism and body composition associated with the aging process itself, and any combination of these factors. In addition to personal contributors to undernutrition, a number of institutional barriers also contribute to undernutrition's incidence and prevalence. These include factors such as a lack of routinely implemented nutrition screening/assessment protocols, failure to recognize undernutrition, failure to provide nutrition intervention to undernourished patients in a timely/coordinated manner, confusion regarding "ownership" of the nutrition screening, assessment, and intervention process, failure to measure or monitor body weight and/or food and nutrient intake, lack of feeding assistance, and low priority given to nutrition status in institutional settings [11, 12].

Clearly, there may be marked variability in the impact of nutrition among patients with different stages of disease, or even different treatments (e.g., chemotherapy, radiotherapy, advanced disease, serious comorbidities, and emergency surgery). However, patients who are malnourished have compromised immunity and are at significantly higher risk for developing SSI. The provision of nutrition support to patients before surgery has been shown to be effective in reducing SSI among surgical colorectal cancer patients [13, 14, 15].

Malnutrition is a major contributor to increased morbidity and mortality, decreased function and quality of life, increased frequency and length of hospital stay, and higher health care costs [16].

NUTRITIONAL SCREENING

Nutrition screening is only the initial step in the identification of patients who are malnourished or at risk to develop. Effective nutritional screening tools should be easy to use, valid and reliable. The screening process should be performed by trained personnel (medical or other health personnel). The Joint Commission on Accreditation of Healthcare Organizations (JCAHO) now mandates that all hospitals conduct nutrition screening within 24 hours of hospital admission [17, 18].

Nutrition assessments may lead to recommendations for improving nutrition status (e.g., some intervention such as change in diet, enteral or parenteral nutrition, or further medical assessment) or a recommendation for re-screening. Unfortunately, nutritional screening and his interventions are inadequate and infrequent. This is reflected in the fact that only 1 in 5 hospitals have formal nutrition screening, also only 1 out of 5 patients receives any preoperative nutrition intervention, therefore is urgently necessary training personnel and implement multidisciplinary teams [19, 20].

In the clinical and research practice BMI (Body mass index) is the most commonly used marker of nutritional status. However, BMI and weight do not alone provide enough information in terms of assessment of nutritional deficit and sarcopenia [21].

There are several tools to nutrition screening with established reliability and validity, each with specific anthropometric and/or diet related criteria measurements, and are appropriate for use in the acute care or medical-surgical adult patient population:

- Nutrition Risk Screening 2002 (NRS-2002)
- Malnutrition Screening Tool (MST)
- Malnutrition Universal Screening Tool (MUST)
- Nutrition Screening Tool (NST)
- PONS (perioperative nutrition screen) score [20]

There is not universal consensus that what tool is the best. however, the European guidelines recommend the Malnutrition Universal Screening Tool (MUST) for the nutritional evaluation of adults in the community; Nutritional Risk Screening 2002 (NRS-2002) for the detection of undernutrition and the risk of its development in hospital settings and Mini-Nutritional Assessment (MNA) for elderly patients in home-care programs, nursing homes and hospitals. No one of before mentioned test except PONS has been specifically designed for use in the perioperative period [22, 23].

The NRS-2002 and Nutrition Risk in Critically ill (NUTRIC) tools are recommended for use in critically ill adult patients due to their ability to account for nutrition status in relation to disease severity [24].

Recently, American Society for Enhanced Recovery (ASER) and Perioperative Quality Initiative (POQI) conducted an extensive literature review and developed and proposed a novel perioperative nutrition screen—the PONS score (perioperative nutrition screen (PONS)). The PONS is a modified version of the Malnutrition Universal Screening Tool (MUST) that has been modified for perioperative use. The PONS determines the presence of nutrition risk based on a patient's BMI, recent changes in weight, reported recent decrease in dietary intake, and preoperative albumin level. In addition, the PONS includes evaluation of preoperative albumin level, as this is a predictor of postoperative complications, including morbidity/mortality [20].

Nutritional Preoperative Interventions

Nutrition support intervention in patients identified by screening and assessment as at risk for malnutrition or malnourished may improve clinical outcomes. Nutrition intervention in malnourished patients was associated with improved nutrition status, nutrient intake, physical function, and quality of life. In addition, hospital readmissions were reduced. Considering the high prevalence of malnutrition and its repercussions in patient morbidity-mortality and healthcare cost, nutritional screening measures must be included in an integrated nutritional care plan for patients while in the hospital. PONS score has been specifically designed for use in perioperative period is the reason that we recommend to implement this screening tool in surgical patients [6, 19, 20].

- PONS questions for clinic-based perioperative nutrition screening
- Does the patient have a low BMI <18.5 kg/m2 (<20 in >65 y of age)?
- Has the patient experienced a weight loss >10% in past 6 months?

- Has the patient had a reduced oral intake by >50% in the past week? (and/or)
- Does the patient have a preoperative serum albumin <3.0 g/dL?

According to the PONS score subdivide patient in two categories:

Nutrition Pathway in Low Nutrition Risk Perioperative Patients (i.e., PONS < 1 and Albumin [ALB] > 3.0)

Patients should be encouraged to take in healthy high-protein (with high-quality protein sources, such as eggs, fish, and lean meats/dairy) complex carbohydrate-rich diets preoperatively. However, many patients will not be able to meet optimal suggested perioperative energy goals of 25 kcal/kg/d and 1.5–2 g/kg/d of protein (~1 g/pound of ideal/adjusted body weight) from routine food intake. Thus, we encourage patients to take high-protein ONSs (oral nutritional supplements) or IMN (immunonutrition) during the perioperative period unrelated to nutritional status [20, 25, 26].

Nutrition Pathway in Patients Found to Be at Nutrition Risk (i.e., PONS > 1 or ALB < 3.0)

In patients found to be at nutrition risk, we recommend high-protein ONS or IMN be given before surgery. This should have a goal of delivering at least 1.2 g/kg/d total of protein. It is the consensus of the group that high-protein ONS should contain >18 g/protein/serving in a balanced formula. A reasonable goal for most patients is 3 high-protein ONS servings per day. Previous data use preoperative ONS demonstrated benefits on the reduction of surgical-site infections in selected weight-losing patients. Again, because many patients do not meet their energy needs from normal food, especially malnourished patients, it is the consensus of this consensus group to encourage the use of high-protein

ONS or IMN. As patient compliance with ONS intake (2–3× a day) is essential for benefit, it is vital to emphasize the key role of ONS in preoperative therapy. Further, cost-effectiveness of ONS in hospitalized patients has been shown in a recent large systematic review [27, 28, 29].

In this context, there are some meta-analyses showed that a multiple nutrient-enhanced nutritional formula (arginine, glutamine, omega 3, fatty acids, nucleotides) was associated with significantly reduced SSI incidence compared with a standard formula, both in the RCTs, however the quality of the evidence was rated very low. Regarding the use of nutritional supplements enhanced with a single nutrient (either arginine, glycine, or branched chain amino acids) with standard nutrition, meta-analyses showed no difference in the risk of SSI although the quality of evidence was low. Notwithstanding, WHO recommends that multiple nutrient enhanced formulas can be used to prevent SSIs in adult patients undergoing major surgery, nevertheless some factors could be considered such as resources and product availability should be carefully assessed, particularly in settings with limited resources [30].

In addition, there are some recommendations that could be adopted according to the Perioperative Quality Initiative (POQI) [20, 30].

Is recommended that patients who are screened as being at nutritional risk before major surgery receive preoperative ONSs for a period of at least seven days. This may be achieved with either of the following:

- IMN formulas (containing arginine and fish oil)
- High-protein ONS (2–3× a day, minimum of 18g protein/dose)

Is recommended that for patients who are screened as being at nutritional risk before major surgery, where oral nutrition supplementation via ONS is not possible, that a dietician be consulted and an enteral feeding tube be placed and home EN (enteral nutrition) initiated for a period of at least seven days. If neither oral nutrition supplementation via ONS nor EN is possible, or when protein/kcal requirement (>50% of recommended intake) cannot be adequately met by ONS/EN, we recommend preoperative PN (parenteral nutrition) to improve outcomes. Is recommend preoperative fasting from midnight be abandoned. Patients undergoing surgery who are considered to have minimal specific risk of aspiration, we encourage unrestricted access to solids for up to 8h before anesthesia and clear fluids for oral intake up to two hours before the induction of anesthesia.

Is recommend a preoperative carbohydrate drink containing at least 45g of carbohydrate to improve insulin sensitivity (except in type I diabetics due to their insulin deficiency state). We suggest that complex carbohydrate (e.g., maltodextrin) be used when available [31].

NUTRITIONAL POSTOPERATIVE INTERVENTIONS

Postoperative nutritional support is vital in maintaining nutritional status during the catabolic postoperative period and underscored by evidence for early and sustained feeding after surgery as part of ERPs (enhanced recovery pathways) protocols [32].

There are some recommendations that could be adopted according to the Perioperative Quality Initiative (POQI) [20].

Is recommend that a high-protein diet (via diet or high-protein ONS) be initiated on the day of surgery in most cases, with exception of patients without bowel in continuity, with bowel ischemia, or persistent bowel obstruction. Traditional "clear liquid" and "full liquid" diets should not be routinely used.

Is recommend reaching an overall protein intake goal is more important than total calorie intake in the postoperative period.

It is recommended standardized protocols for postoperative nutrition support be instituted.

IMN should be considered in all postoperative major abdominal surgical patients for at least 7 days.

In patients who meet criteria for malnutrition, who are not anticipated to meet nutritional goals (>50% of protein/kcal) through oral intake, we recommend early EN or tube feeding within 24 h. Where goals are not met through EN, we recommend early PN, in combination with EN if possible.

Is recommend when using gastric residual volume's as a marker of feeding tolerance, a cutoff of >500 mL should be used before the tube feeds being suspended or tube feed/EN rate reduced.

In patients started on EN and/or PN, we recommend continuation of EN or PN support for patients who are not able to take in at least 60% of their protein/kcal requirements via the oral route.

Is recommend posthospital high-protein ONS in all patients after major surgery to meet both calorie and protein needs, especially in the previously malnourished, elderly and sarcopenic patient.

NUTRITION IN ILL CRITRICAL PATIENTS

Nutritional support during critical illness attenuates the metabolic response to stress, prevents oxidative cellular injury, and modulates the immune system. The stress response to critical illness causes wide fluctuation in metabolic rate.

The hyper-catabolic phase can last for 7–10 days and is manifested by an increase in oxygen demands, cardiac output, and carbon dioxide production. Caloric needs may be increased by up to 100% during this phase. The goal is to provide ongoing monitoring and support with high-protein feedings while avoiding overfeeding and underfeeding. Nutritional modulation of the stress response includes early EN (enteral nutrition), appropriate macro-nutrient and micro-nutrient delivery, and glycemic control [33].

Primary goals of nutritional support and care are to: Preserve and maintain lean muscle mass, provide continuous assessment, reassessment, and modification to optimize outcome, monitor the patient for tolerance and complications such as refeeding syndrome, prevent protein energy malnutrition by giving higher protein content while providing adequate total calories; monitor nutrition goals and target achievement rate of >50%

within the first week, and prevent accumulation of a caloric deficit. Indirect calorimetry should be used when available or when predictive equations are known to be inaccurate [33].

The Society of Critical Care Medicine and the American Society of Parenteral and Enteral Nutrition (SCCM/ASPEN), the European Society for Clinical Nutrition and Metabolism (ESPEN), the Academy of Nutrition and Dietetics (AND), and the Canadian Clinical Practice Guidelines for Nutritional Support (CCPG) have developed best practice recommendations:

Nutritional support should be initiated early within the first 24–48 hours in critically ill patients. Current EN practice recommendations are: Preferentially feed via the enteral route, initiate EN within 24–48 hours, reduce interruptions of EN for nursing care and bedside procedures to prevent underfeeding, maintain head of bed (HOB) elevation to reduce aspiration risk, accept GRV (Gastric Residual Volume) up to 500 mL before reducing or stopping EN in the absence of clear signs of intolerance, use motility agents to improve tolerance and reduce GRV, and promote post-pyloric feeding tube placement when feasible. Current PN (Parenteral Nutrition) practice recommendations are to: Only use PN when enteral route is not feasible, use PN based on the patient's nutritional risk classification for malnutrition, delay PN up to seven days if the patient is in Nutritional Risk Class I or II, initiate PN early if the patient is in Nutritional Risk Class III or IV, convert to EN as soon as tolerated to reduce the risks associated with PN. Use of trophic or "trickle feeding" and permissive underfeeding may be beneficial [33, 35].

Use of pharmaconutrients and immunonutrition: Omega-3 fatty acids (fish oils) may be beneficial in acute respiratory distress syndrome (ARDS) patients, use high omega-3 fatty acid to omega-6 fatty acid ratios. The use of arginine, glutamine, nucleotides, antioxidants, and probiotics may be beneficial in specific patients. The use of arginine should be avoided in patients with severe sepsis [36].

REFERENCES

[1] Allegranzi B, Bagheri Nejad S, Combescure C, et al. Burden of endemic health-care-associated infection in developing countries: systematic review and meta-analysis. *Lancet* 2011.
[2] WHO. *Report on the burden of endemic health care-associated infection worldwide*. Geneva: World Health Organization, 2011.
[3] Horan TC, Gaynes RP, Martone WJ, et al. CDC definitions of nosocomial surgical site infections, 1992: a modification of CDC definitions of surgical wound infections. *Am J Infect Control* 1992; 20:271.
[4] Nolan MB, Martin DP, Thompson R, et al. Association Between Smoking Status, Preoperative Exhaled Carbon Monoxide Levels, and Postoperative Surgical Site Infection in Patients Undergoing Elective Surgery. *JAMA Surg* 2017; 152:476.
[5] Hennessey DB, Burke JP, Ni-Dhonochu T, et al. Preoperative hypoalbuminemia is an independent risk factor for the development of surgical site infection following gastrointestinal surgery: a multi-institutional study. *Ann Surg 2010*; 252:325.
[6] Culebras JM. Malnutrition in the twenty-first century: an epidemic affecting surgical outcome. *Surg Infect (Larchmt)* 2013, 14: 237–43.
[7] Bernabeu-Wittel M, Jadad A, Moreno-Gavino L, et al. Peeking through the cracks: an assessment of the prevalence, clinical characteristics and health-related quality of life (HRQoL) of people with polypathology in a hospital setting. *Arch Gerontol Geriatr* 2009.
[8] Edington J, Boorman J, Durrant ER, et al. The Malnutrition Prevalence Group. Prevalence of malnutrition on admission to four hospitals in England. *Clin Nutr* 2000; 19(3):191–195.
[9] Rasmussen HH, Kondrup J, Staun M, Ladefoged K, Kristensen H, Wengler A. Prevalence of patients at nutritional risk in Danish hospitals. *Clin Nutr 2004*; 23(5):1009–1015.
[10] Malone A, Hamilton C. The Academy of Nutrition and Dietetics/The American Society for Parenteral and Enteral Nutrition [ASPEN]

consensus malnutrition characteristics: Application in practice. *Nutrition clinical practice. 2013*; 28(6), 639-650.

[11] White J, Stotts N, Jones S, Granieri, E. Managing post acute malnutrition (undernutrition) risk. *Journal of parenteral and enteral nutrition* 2013; 37(6), 816-823.

[12] Barker LA, Gout BS, Crowe TC. Hospital malnutrition: prevalence, identification and impact on patients and the healthcare system. *Int J Environ Res Public Health*. 2011;8(2):514-527.

[13] Brigid MG, Evelyn K, Shelley R, Reducing the risk of surgical site infection using a multidisciplinary approach: an integrative review. *J Multidisciplinary Healthcare* 2015; 8: 473–487.

[14] Schneider SM, Veyres P, Pivot X, et al. Malnutrition is an independent factor associated with nosocomial infections. *Br J Nutr* 2004;92(1):105–111.

[15] Horie H, Okada M, Kojima M, Nagai H. Favorable effects of preoperative enteral immunonutrition on a surgical site infection in patients with colorectal cancer without malnutrition. *Surg Today* 2006;36(12):1063–1068.

[16] National Alliance for Infusion Therapy and the American Society for Parenteral and Enteral Nutrition Public Policy Committee and Board of Directors. Disease-related malnutrition and enteral nutrition therapy: a significant problem with a cost-effective solution. *Nutr Clin Pract* 2010; 25:548-554.

[17] Skipper A, Ferguson M, Thompson K, Castellanos V. Nutrition Screening Tools an Analysis of the Evidence. *Journal of Parenteral and Enteral Nutrition* 2012; 36(3), 292-298.

[18] Joint Commission on Accreditation of Healthcare Organizations. *Comprehensive Accreditation Manual for Hospitals*. Oakbrook Terrace, IL: *JCAHO*; 2005.

[19] Charles M, Charlene C, et al. A. S. P. E. N. Clinical Guidelines Nutrition Screening, Assessment, and Intervention in Adults. *Journal of Parenteral and Enteral Nutrition* 2011; 35(1):16-24.

[20] Paul EW, Franco C, David C, et al. American society for enhanced recovery and perioperative quality initiative joint consensus

statement on nutrition screening and therapy within a surgical enhanced recovery pathway. *Anesth Analg 2018*; 126(6):1883-1895.

[21] Kuźnar-Kamińska B, Batura-Gabryel H, Brajer B, Kamiński J. Analysis of nutritional status disorders in patients with chronic obstructive pulmonary disease. *Pneumonol Alergol Pol* 2008; 76(5):327-33.

[22] van Bokhorst-de van der Schueren MA, Guaitoli PR, Jansma EP. Nutrition screening tools: does one size fit all? A systematic review of screening tools for the hospital setting. *Clin Nutr* 2014; 33(1):39-58.

[23] Sorensen J, Kondrup J, Prokopowicz J, Schiesser M, Krahenbuh L, Meier R et al. EuroOOPS study group. EuroOOPS: an international, multicenter study to implement nutritional risk screening and evaluate clinical outcome. *Clin Nutr* 2008; 27: 340–349.

[24] McClave SA, Taylor BE, MartindaleRG, et al. Guidelines for the Provision and Assessment of Nutrition Support Therapy in the Adult Critically Ill Patient Society of Critical Care Medicine (SCCM) and American Society for Parenteral and Enteral Nutrition (ASPEN). *Journal of Parenteral and Enteral Nutrition* 2016; 40(2), 159-211.

[25] Miller KR, Wischmeyer PE, Taylor B, McClave SA. An evidence-based approach to perioperative nutrition support in the elective surgery patient. *J Parenter Enteral* Nutr 2013; 37:39S–50S.

[26] Braga M, Ljungqvist O, Soeters P, Fearon K, Weimann A, Bozzetti F. ESPEN guidelines on parenteral nutrition: surgery. *Clin Nutr* 2009; 28:378–386.

[27] Grass F, Bertrand PC, Schäfer M, et al. Compliance with preoperative oral nutritional supplements in patients at nutritional risk—only a question of will? *Eur J Clin Nutr* 2015; 69:525–529.

[28] Elia M, Normand C, Norman K, Laviano A. A systematic review of the cost and cost effectiveness of using standard oral nutritional supplements in the hospital setting. *Clin Nutr* 2016; 35:370–380.

[29] Fukuda Y, Yamamoto K, Hirao M, et al. Prevalence of malnutrition among gastric cancer patients undergoing gastrectomy andoptimal

preoperative nutritional support for preventing surgical site infections. *Ann Surg Oncol* 2015;22(suppl 3): S778–S785.

[30] WHO. *Gobal guidelines for the prevention of surgical site infections.* World Health Organization, Geneva, 2016.

[31] Harbis A, Perdreau S, Vincent-Baudry S, et al. Glycemic and insulinemic meal responses modulate postprandial hepatic and intestinal lipoprotein accumulation in obese, insulin-resistant subjects. *Am J Clin Nutr 2004*; 80:896–902.

[32] Osland E, Yunus RM, Khan S, Memon MA. Early versus traditional postoperative feeding in patients undergoing resectional gastrointestinal surgery: a meta-analysis. *JPEN J Parenter Enteral Nutr* 2011; 35:473–487.

[33] Mark S. Siobal, Jami E. Baltz. *A Guide to the Nutritional Assessment and Treatment of the Critically Ill Patient.* American association for respiratory care 2013, 007-029.

[34] Rice TW, Wheeler AP, Thompson BT, et al. Initial trophic vs full enteral feeding in patients with acute lung injury: the EDEN randomized trial. *JAMA* 2012; 307(8):795-803.

[35] Poulard F, Dimet J, Martin-Lefevre L, et al. Impact of not measuring residual gastric volume in mechanically ventilated patients receiving early enteral feeding: a prospective before-after study. *J Parenter Enteral Nutr* 2010; 34(2):125-130.

[36] Marik PE, Zaloga GP. Immunonutrition in high-risk surgical patients: a systematic review and analysis of the literature. *J Parenter Enteral Nutr* 2010; 34(4):378-386.

In: Prophylaxis of Surgical Site Infection … ISBN: 978-1-53615-615-7
Editors: Jaime Ruiz-Tovar et al. © 2019 Nova Science Publishers, Inc.

Chapter 3

PREOPERATIVE BATH AND SHAVE

Cristina Bernabeu Herraiz[*], MD*
and Lorena Rodríguez Cazalla, MD
Department of General and Digestive Surgery,
University Hospital San Juan,
Alicante, Spain

ABSTRACT

Surgical site infection is one of the most common complication in surgery, that increases length of hospital stay and health cost. This chapter is focused on preoperative bath and hair removal. There is neither clear evidence about the benefits to reduce surgical site infection for preoperative showering or bathing with chlorhexidine nor routine hair removal, which should be performed if it is necessary with clippers instead of razors.

Keywords: surgical site infection, preoperative bath and shower, skin antiseptics, preoperative hair removal

---

[*] Corresponding Author's Email: cristina.bernabeu.h@gmail.com.

INTRODUCTION

Surgical site infection (SSI) is a major problem for patients undergoing surgery because it increases not only the cost of health care related to a need of antibiotic therapy and a higher length of hospital stay, but also affects patient recovery [1, 2]. Surgeons and health care authorities pay attention to prevent SSI, since up to 60% of them are avoidable applying adequate prevention programs [1-3].

This chapter is focused on preoperative showering or bathing and hair removal.

PREOPERATIVE BATH

Whole body bathing or showering with soap or skin antiseptics is a widespread practice before surgery to reduce skin resident and transient bacteria. However the most important question is whether preoperative bathing or showering with antiseptics reduce the incidence of SSI in comparison with their potential for harm such as changes in patterns of bacteria resistance, skin hipersensitivity, etc.

Webster and Osborne reviewed randomized clinical trials comparing antiseptic preparation (4% chlorhexidine gluconate) for preoperative bathing or showering with non-antiseptic preparations or no washing over a 26-year period between 1983 and 2009 (seven trials with 10.157 participants). Three trials involving 7.791 patients compared chlorhexidine with placebo did not result in a significant reduction in SSI with a relative risk of 0.91 (0.80 - 1.04). Three trials involving 1.443 patients compared bar soap with chlorhexidine and there was no significant differences with a relative risk of 1.02 (0.57 - 1.84) and three trials of 1.192 patients compared bathing with chlorhexidine with no washing and only one found a significant difference in favour of bathing with chlorhexidine (relative risk 0.36 [0.17 - 0.79]. Authors concluded that this review does not provide clear evidence of benefit for preoperative showering or bathing with chlorhexidine over other wash products to reduce SSI [4]. Smaller studies have not found differences between patients who washed with chlorhexidine and those who did not wash preoperatively [5-7].

Chlebicki et al. performed a meta-analysis of sixteen trials involving 17.932 patients, 7.952 received a chlorhexidine bath and 9.980 with others. Chlorhexidine bathing did not significantly reduce overal incidence of SSI when compared with soap, placebo or no shower or bath (relative risk 0.90 [0.77 - 1.05]) [8].

PREOPERATIVE SHAVE

Preparation the patient for surgery has traditionally included the routine hair removal from the incision site because its presence can interfere with the exposure, the suturing and the application of adhesive drapes. However some studies claim that preoperative hair removal is harmful, increase SSI and should be avoided [9, 10].

Hair can be removed by several different ways which include shaving, clipping the hair and using a chemical creams. Shaving is the commonest and cheapest method, it uses a sharp blade, which is drawn over the patient's skin to cut hair close to the surface of the skin. Clippers use fine teeth to cut hair close to the patient's skin, leaving around one millimetre of hair in length. Depilatory creams are chemicals which dissolve the hair itself, but is a slower process, because the cream has to remain in contact with the hair for between five and 20 minutes, that's why there is a risk of irritant or allergic reactions to the cream. During the process of shaving, the skin may experience microscopic cuts and abrasions. It is believed that microorganisms are able to colonize these cuts, thus contaminating the surgical incision site and causing wound infections. That's why clippers they are thought to reduce the risk of cuts and abrasions because do not come into contact with the patient's skin. This hair removal practice can be done everywhere (home, wards, theaters...) but research has suggested, that hair removal should not take place in the operating theatre as loose hair may contaminate the sterile surgical field [11].

Tanner et al. performed a meta-analysis of fourteen trials; six trials compared hair removal (shaving, clipping or depilatory cream) with no hair removal and found no statistically significant difference in SSI rates. Three trials that compared shaving with clipping showed significantly more SSI associated with shaving (relative risk 2.09 [1.15 - 3.80]. Seven trials found no significant difference in SSI rate when hair removal by shaving was compared with depilatory cream (relative risk 1.53 [0.73 - 3.21]. One trial compared two groups that shaved or clipped hair on the day of surgery compared with the day before surgery and there was no statistically significant difference in SSI rate. Authors concluded that there was no significantly differences between hair removal and not hair removal; however, when it is necessary to remove hair, the evidence suggests that clippers are associated with fewer SSI than razors [9].

Lefebvre et al. performed a meta-analysis of nineteen randomized controlled trials and they described no significant differences between the absence of hair removal and chemical depilation (relative risk 1.05 [0.55 - 2.00]) or clipping (relative risk 0.97 [0.51 - 1.82]) as well as a higher significantly risk of SSI when shaving is used for hair removal in comparison with clipping (relative risk 0.55 [0.38 - 0.79], chemical depilation (relative risk 0.60 [0.36 - 0.97] or no depilation (relative risk 0.56 [0.34 - 0.96]) [12].

Kowalski et al. conducted a single-center randomized clinical trial, 834 patients to clipped group and 844 to not-clipped group. The overall rate of SSI in the per-protocol analysis was 6.12% in clipped group and 6.32% in not-clipped group (absolute risk difference -0.20 [-2.61 to 2.21%]). Authors concluded that SSI rate was similar between hair removal by clipping or not in patients undergoing general surgical procedures [13].

REFERENCES

[1] World Health Organization. *Global Guidelines for the Prevention of Surgical Site Infection.* Geneva: WHO; 2016.

[2] Gómez-Romero, F. J., Fernández-Prada, M., Navarro-Gracia, J. F. Prevention of Surgical Site Infection; analysis and narrative. Review of Clinical Practice Guidelines. *Cir. Esp.*, 2017; 95(9):490 - 502.

[3] EPINE Wordkgroup. *EPINE-EPPS 2017 Study. Spanish Society of Preventive Medicine, Public Health and Hygiene* [Internet]. Available at: http://hws.vhebron.net/epine/Global/EPINE-EPPS%20 2017%20Informe%20Global%20de%20España%20Resumen.pdf.

[4] Webster, J., Osborne, S. Preoperative bathing or showering with skin antiseptics to prevent surgical site infection. *Cochrane Database of Systematic Reviews,* 2015, Issue 2. Art. No.: CD004985. DOI: 10.1002/14651858.CD004985.pub5.

[5] Kamel, C., McGahan, L., Polisina, J., Miezwinski-Urban, M., Embil, J. M. Preoperative skin antiseptic preparations for preventing surgical site infections: a systematic review. *Infect. Control Hosp. Epidemiol.,* 2012; 33(6):608 - 617.

[6] Thomas, L., Maillard, J. Y., Lambert, R. J., Russell, A. D. Development of resistance to chlorhexidine diacetate in Pseudomonas aeruginosa and the effect of a "residual" concentration. *J. Hosp. Infect.,* 2000; 46(4):297 - 304.

[7] Chlebicki, M. P., Safdar, N., O'Horo, J. C., Maki, D. G. Preoperative chlorhexidine shower of bath for prevention of surgical site infection: a meta-analysis. *Am. J. Infect. Control.,* 2013; 41(2):167 - 173.

[8] Chlebicki, M. P., Safdar, N., O'Horo, J. C., Maki, D. G. Preoperative chlorhexidine shower of bath for prevention of surgical site infection: a meta-analysis. *Am. J. Infect. Control.,* 2013; 41(2):167 - 173.

[9] Tanner, J., Norrie, P., Melen, K. Preoperative hair removal to reduce surgical site infection. *Cochrane Database of Systematic Reviews,* 2011, Issue 11. Art. No.: CD004122. DOI: 10.1002/ 14651858.CD004122.pub4.

[10] Ruiz-Tovar, J., Badia, J. M. Prevention of surgical site infection in abdominal surgery. A critical review of the evidence. *Cir. Esp.,* 2014; 92(4):223 - 231.

[11] Phippen, M., Papanier, M. *Patient care during operative and invasive procedures.* Philadelphia: WB Saunders Co, 2000.

[12] Lefebvre, A., Saliou, P., Lucet, J. C., Mimoz, O., Keita-Perse, O., Grandbastien, B., et al. Preoperative hair removal and surgical site infections: network meta-analysis of randomized controlled trials. *J. Hosp. Infect.,* 2015; 91(2):100 - 108.

[13] Kowalski, T. J., Kothari, S. N., Mathiason, M. A., Borgert, A. J. Impact of hair removal on surgical site infection rates: a prospective randomized noninferiority trial. *J. Am. Coll. Surg.,* 2016; 223(5):704 - 711.

In: Prophylaxis of Surgical Site Infection …   ISBN: 978-1-53615-615-7
Editors: Jaime Ruiz-Tovar et al.   © 2019 Nova Science Publishers, Inc.

Chapter 4

MECHANICAL BOWEL PREPARATION

*Andrés García Marín,[1] MD, PhD
and Mercedes Pérez López[2],**

[1]Department of General and Digestive Surgery,
Hospital Hellín, Albacete, Spain
[2]Department of Nursery,
Alicante, Spain

ABSTRACT

The chapter summarizes the recent evidence about the role of mechanical bowel preparation in combination with oral antibiotic prophylaxis in comparison with No Preparation or mechanical bowel preparation alone in the prevention of postoperative morbidity, surgical site infection, anastomotic leakage and ileus, mortality rate and *Clostridium difficile* infection.

Keywords: mechanical bowel preparation, oral antibiotic prophylaxis, surgical site infection, anastomotic leakage, ileus, colorectal surgery, mortality

---

* Mercedes Pérez López, RN.

INTRODUCTION

Surgical site infection (SSI) is a major problem for patients undergoing colorectal surgery (CRS) because it increases not only the cost of health care related to a need of antibiotic therapy and a higher length of hospital stay, but also affects patient recovery and survival [1-3].

Mechanical bowel preparation (MBP) and oral antibiotic prophylaxis (OAP) are specific strategies to prevent SSI in CRS.

MBP defined as oral preparations prior to surgery to clear out solid stool has been studied in randomized controlled trials (RCT). Rollins et al. concluded in a recent meta-analysis of 36 RCT that MBP does not impact in postoperative morbidity and mortality, as well as it produces fluid and electrolyte disturbances and patient dissatisfaction [2, 4].

In fact, Enhanced Recovery After Surgery Society and the American Society for Enhanced Recovery do not recommend the use of MBP without OAP before elective CRS [5, 6].

OAP with nonabsorbable luminal antibiotics, mainly the combination of an aminoglycoside (neomycin or kanamycin) with erythromycin or metronidazole, was firstly proposed in 1971 by Rosenberg and Nichols [7, 8].

Table 1. Comparison between MBP + OAP and MBP alone, No Preparation and OAP [2]

	Studies	RR (95% CI)
30-day mortality		
MBP + OAP vs MBP	17 (14 RCT and 3 CS)	0.58 (0.44-0.76)
MBP + OAP vs No Preparation	2 CS	0.36 (0.17-0.76)
MBP + OAP vs OAP	3 (2 RCT and 1 CS)	0.58 (0.34-0.97)

CS: Cohort Studies. MBP: Mechanical Bowel Preparation. OAP: Oral Antibiotic Prophylaxis. RCT: Randomized Clinical Trial. RR (95% CI): relative risk (95% confidence interval).

RECENT EVIDENCE

Overall, the combination of MBP + OAP is associated with a significant reduction in global morbidity, SSI, anastomotic leakage, postoperative ileus and 30-day mortality in comparison with MBP alone, No Preparation and OAP alone [1, 2, 9-14].

A summary of the evidence related to 30-day mortality is presented in table 1, and related to SSI (table 2), anastomotic leakage (AL) and postoperative ileus in table 3.

The value of different regimens of oral antibiotics is being evaluated. McSorley et al. conducted a meta-analysis and they concluded that there was a similarly significant effect on SSI with the use of a combination of aminoglycoside and erythromycin (OR 0.40 [0.25 - 0.64]) or aminoglycoside and metronidazole (OR 0.51 [0.39 - 0.68]) [1].

Evidence about *Clostridium difficile* infection was enough for the comparison between MBP + OAP versus MBP in 14 studies (10 RCT and 4 cohort studies), without significant differences (RR 0.94 [0.55 - 1.61]) [2].

Table 2. Comparison between MBP + OAP and MBP alone, NP and OAP [2]

	Studies	RR (95% CI)
SSI		
MBP + OAP vs MBP	35 (26 RCT and 9 CS)	0.51 (0.46-0.56)
MBP + OAP vs NP	4 CS	0.54 (0.43-0.68)
MBP + OAP vs OAP	4 (2 RCT and 2 CS)	0.98 (0.64-1.50)
MBP + OAP vs MBP in laparoscopic vs open approach	Open: 19 RCT. Laparoscopic: 2 RCT	Open: 0.55 (0.44-0.69) Laparoscopic: 0.74 (0.43-1.29)

CS: Cohort Studies. MBP: Mechanical Bowel Preparation. NP: No Preparation. OAP: Oral Antibiotic Prophylaxis. RCT: Randomized Clinical Trial. RR (95% CI): relative risk (95% confidence interval). SSI: Surgical Site Infection.

Table 3. Comparison between MBP + OAP and MBP alone, NP and OAP [2]

AL		
MBP + OAP vs MBP	22 (17 RCT and 5 CS)	0.62 (0.55-0.70)
MBP + OAP vs NP	2 CS	0.52 (0.45-0.59)
MBP + OAP vs OAP	3 (2 RCT and 1 CS)	0.79 (0.59-1.05)
MBP + OAP vs MBP in laparoscopic vs open approach	Open: 9 RCT. Laparoscopic: 2 RCT	Open: 0.69 (0.30-1.60) Laparoscopic: 0.68 (0.28-1.65)
Ileus		
MBP + OAP vs MBP	5 (2 RCT and 3 CS)	0.72 (0.52-0.98)
MBP + OAP vs NP	2 CS	0.72 (0.68-0.77)
MBP + OAP vs OAP	3 (2 RCT + 1 CS)	0.83 (0.73-0.95)
Overall morbidity		
MBP + OAP vs MBP	6 (4 RCT + 2 CS)	0.67 (0.63-0.71)

AL: Anastomotic Leakage. CS: Cohort Studies. MBP: Mechanical Bowel Preparation. NP: No Preparation. OAP: Oral Antibiotic Prophylaxis. RCT: Randomized Clinical Trial. RR (95% CI): relative risk (95% confidence interval).

CONCLUSION

The combination of MBP and OAP was associated with a significant reduction in overall morbidity, SSI, AL, ileus and 30-day mortality in comparison with MBP alone and No Preparation and only in ileus and 30-day mortality in comparison with OAP alone. However, there was not significant differences in *Clostridium difficile* infection.

REFERENCES

[1] McSorley, S. T., Steele, C. W., McMahon, A. J. Meta-analysis of oral antibiotics, in combination with preoperative intravenous antibiotics

and mechanical bowel preparation the day before surgery, compared with intravenous antibiotics and mechanical bowel preparation alone to reduce surgical-site infections in elective colorectal surgery. *BJS Open,* 2018; 2:185 - 194.

[2] Rollins, K. E., Javanmard-Emamghissi, H., Acheson, A. G., Lobo, D. N. The role of oral antibiotic preparation in elective colorectal surgery: a meta-analysis. *Ann. Surg.,* 2018 Dec. 3 [Epub ahead of print].

[3] Badia, J. M., Arroyo-García, N. Mechanical bowel preparation and oral antibiotic prophylaxis in colorectal surgery: analysis of evidence and narrative review. *Cir. Esp.,* 2018; 96(6):317 - 325.

[4] Rollins, K. E., Javanmard-Emamghissi, H., Lobo, D. N. Impact of mechanical preparation in elective colorectal surgery: a meta-analysis. *World J. Gastroenterol.,* 2018; 24(4):519 - 536.

[5] Gustafsson, U. O., Scott, M. J., Schwenk, W., Demartines, N., Roulin, D., Francis, N., et al. Guidelines for perioperative care in elective colonic surgery: Enhanced Recovery After Surgery (ERAS®) Society recommendations. *Clin. Nutr.,* 2012; 31(6):783 - 800.

[6] Holubar, S. D., Hedrick, T., Gupta, R., Kellum, J., Hamilton, M., Gan, T. J., et al. American Society for Enhanced Recovery (ASER) and Perioperative Quality Initiative (POQI) joint consensus statement on prevention of postoperative infection within an enhanced recovery pathway for elective colorectal surgery. *Perioper. Med.,* (Lond) [Internet] 2017; 4. Available at: https://www.ncbi.nlm.nih.gov/pmc/articles/PMC5335800/pdf/13741_2017_Article_59.pdf.

[7] Rosenberg, I. L., Graham, N. G., De Dombal, F. T., Goligher, J. C. Preparation of the intestine in patients undergoing major large-bowel surgery, mainly for neoplasms of the colon and rectum. *Br. J. Surg.,* 1971; 58(4):266 - 269.

[8] Nichols, R. L., Condon, R. E. *Preoperative preparation of the colon Surg. Gynecol. Obstet.,* 1971; 132 (2):323 - 337.

[9] Yost, M. T., Jolissaint, J. S., Fields, A. C., Whang, E. E. Mechanical and oral antibiotic bowel preparation in the era of minimally invasive

surgery and enhanced recovery. *J. Laparoendosc. Adv. Surg. Tech. A.*, 2018; 28(5):491 - 495.

[10] Toh, J. W. T., Phan, K., Ctercteko, G., Pathma-Nathan, N., El-Khoury, T., Richardson, A., et al. The role of mechanical bowel preparation and oral antibiotics for left-sided laparoscopic and open elective restorative colorectal surgery with and without faecal diversion. *Int. J. Colorectal. Dis.*, 2018; 33(12):1781 - 1791.

[11] Ohman, K. A., Wan, L., Guthrie, T., Johnston, B., Leinicke, J. A., Glasgow, S. C., et al. Combination of oral antibiotics and mechanical bowel preparation reduces surgical site infection in colorectal surgery. *J. Am. Coll. Surg.*, 2017; 225(4):465 - 471.

[12] Chen, M., Song, X., Chen, L. Z., Lin, Z. D., Zhang, X. L. Comparing mechanical bowel preparation with both oral and systemic antibiotics versus mechanical bowel preparation and systemic antibiotics alone for the prevention of surgical site infection after elective colorectal surgery: a meta-analysis of randomized controlled clinical trials. *Dis. Colon Rectum*, 2016; 59(1):70 - 78.

[13] Ambe, P. C., Zarras, K., Stodolski, M., Wirjawan, I., Zirngibl, H. Routine preoperative mechanical bowel preparation with additive oral antibiotics is associated with a reduced risk of anastomotic leakage in patients undergoing elective oncologic resection for colorectal cancer. *World J. Surg. Oncol.*, [Internet] 2019; 17. Available at: https://www.ncbi.nlm.nih.gov/pmc/articles/ PMC633 5695/pdf/12957_2019_Article_1563.pdf.

[14] Battersby, C. L. F., Battersby, N. J., Slade, D. A. J., Soop, M., Walsh, C. J. Preoperative mechanical and oral antibiotic bowel preparation to reduce infectious complications of colorectal surgery – the need for updated guidelines. *J. Hosp. Infect.*, 2019; 101(3):295 - 299.

In: Prophylaxis of Surgical Site Infection …   ISBN: 978-1-53615-615-7
Editors: Jaime Ruiz-Tovar et al.   © 2019 Nova Science Publishers, Inc.

Chapter 5

ANTIBIOTIC PROPHYLAXIS

Noel Rojas-Bonet[1,][*] MD, and Maria del Mar García-Navarro[2] MD

[1]Department of General and Digestive Surgery,
University Hospital San Juan, Alicante, Spain
[2]Department of Internal Medicine,
University General Hospital of Alicante,
Alicante, Spain

ABSTRACT

The chapter summarizes the recent evidence about microbiology, indications, recommended antibiotics, timing and dosages in patients undergoing general and digestive procedures.

Keywords: antibiotic prophylaxis, surgical site infection

---

[*] Corresponding Author's Email: noel.rojas@goumh.umh.es.

INTRODUCTION

Surgical site infections (SSI) is defined as infection related to a surgical procedure that occurs within 30 days of the procedure or withing 90 days if prosthetic material is implanted at surgery, which may be incisional (superficial or deep) or organ/space [1].

The goal of antimicrobial prophylaxis is to control bacterial burden, mantaining antibiotic levels above the minimum inhibitory concentration throughout the surgical procedure in order to reduce the risk of infection [1].

EPIDEMIOLOGY

The estimated incidence of SSI ranges from 1% in minimally invasive surgery to 5% in invasive surgery. However, this percentage is probably underestimated, as up to 50% of post-surgical infections occur after discharge [2, 3].

The severity of surgical site infections depends on many factors: type of surgery, surgical technique, bacterial inoculum, responsible organism (as well as mono or polymicrobial) and patient characteristics and comorbidities.

Patient risk factors (modifiable and non-modifiable) can contribute to the development of infections and complications [3].

Risk factors whose presence have been directly related to torpid evolution and higher infection rates of the surgical site are those conferring greater difficulty in healing and therefore will increase the period of vulnerability for the appearance of superinfections: age, smoking, the nutritional status, the immunosuppression both intrinsic (primary immunodeficiency, HIV, cancer...) and extrinsic (corticoids, chemotherapy) that hinders the adequate inflammatory response and the defense against the potential risk of infections, diabetes, obesity, peripheral edema and immobilization [4].

Thus, a relationship is found between the comorbidities of the patients and the prevalence of SSI after invasive surgery (ASA I 1.7%, ASA II 4.1%, ASA III 7.3%, ASA IV 7.9%, ASA V 14.3%) [3, 4].

MICROBIOLOGY

The main involved microorganisms in SSI are those found in the skin, mainly grampositive cocci (*Staphylococcus spp.*, *Streptococcus spp.* and, less frequently, *Enterococcus spp.*) and those found in abdominal cavity, mainly gram-negative bacilli (*Escherichia coli, Proteus spp., Klebsiella spp.*) and anaerobes (*Bacteroides spp.*) [1].

GENERAL PRINCIPLES OF ANTIBIOTIC PROPHYLAXIS

General principles are intravenous administration and selection of adequate antibiotic with correct posology.

The antibiotic should present a narrow spectrum to cover the typical microorganisms, bactericidal actitiy, extended half life, good tissue distribution and low adverse effects including a low rate of *Clostridium difficile* infection. According to this, the recommended antibiotic for surgeries above the duodenum in abdominal cavity, neck and breast surgeries would be cefazolin and, in patients with β-lactam allergies, vancomycin and gentamicin, clindamycin and gentamicin or levofloxacin whereas for surgeries below the duodenum, amoxicillin-clavulanic and, in patients with β-lactam allergies, moxifloxacin, levofloxacin and metronidazole or gentamicin and metronidazole are preferred.

The administration should be performed 30-60 minutes before the start of the procedure; if it is administered more than 120 minutes before, the risk of infection is double that if it is administered in the 120 minutes prior to surgery. If the administration is delayed until after the surgical initiation, the risk of infection is multiplied by 5 [1, 3, 5-9].

Intraoperative redosing is recommended when bleeding greather than 1500 mililiters occurs or surgical procedure lasts more than two half-life of the antibiotic, only for amoxicillin-clavulanic acid at 2-3 hours, cefazolin at 4 hours and clindamycin at 6 hours. Intraoperative redosing is not required for gentamicin / tobramycin, metronidazole and vancomycin [3, 5-9]. Classical administration with redosing is controversial. In fact, Kirby et al. conducted a colorectal study comparing standard bolus-dosed antibiotic with continuous administration throughout surgery monitoring serum antibiotic concentrations and they showed that the rates of SSI were lower with continuous administration [10].

Postoperative redosing in clean and clean-contaminated surgeries is not recommended with high level of evidence once the surgical incision has been closed, even if drainage is required [3, 6, 8].

Dosing adjustment should be performed according to the patient comorbidities and weight, since the alteration in body composition in obese patients involves a higher risk of erroneous dosing and, therefore, a possible therapeutic failure or toxicity [1, 11, 12]:

- Cefazolin and amoxicillin-clavulanic acid (80 - 160kg): 2gr. Patients lower than 80kg. 1gr., whereas the dosage in patients higher than 160kg is controversial (same or high dose of 3 - 4gr).
- Cefuroxime (> 80kg): 3gr. Patients lower than 80kg. 1.5g.
- Gentamicin: 5 - 7mg/kg.
- Vancomycin: 15mg/kg, with maximum dose of 2gr.
- Clindamycin: 600 – 900. In patient with body mass index higher than 50 kg/m2, a high dose of 900 – 1200 is recommended.
- Metronidazole: 15mg/kg.

INDICATIONS

Indications for antibiotic prophylaxis are controversial, depending on the type of surgery. Antibiotic prophylaxis is not always needed for clean surgery since the rate of SSI is very low; it should only be administered in some patients such as oncological and plastic breast surgery, intravascular devices placement, splenectomy in immunosuppression situations and mesh surgery in high risk patients [13-15]. Antibiotic prophylaxis is always needed in clean-contaminated and contaminated procedures; however, it is still unclear in elective laparoscopic cholecystectomy in low-risk patients, considering high risk patients immunosuppressive therapy or disease, ASA ≥ III, acute or chronic cholecystitis 6 weeks before surgery, open conversion surgery or intraoperative rupture of the gallbladder [17-19].

REFERENCES

[1] Garcia-Marin, A., Perez-Lopez, M. Antibiotic Prophylaxis. In: Ruiz-Tovar, J. *Prophylaxis in Bariatric Surgery*. New York: Nova Biomedical, 2018, p. 1 - 7.

[2] *Sociedad Española de Medicina Preventiva, Salud Pública e Higiene* [*Spanish Society of Preventive Medicine, Public Health and Hygiene*] (2017). ESTUDIO EPINE-EPPS 2017. [Internet] Available at: http://hws.vhebron.net/epine/Global/EPINE-EPPS%202017%20 Informe%20Global%20de%20Espa%C3%B1a%20Resumen.pdf.

[3] Berríos-Torres, S. I., Umscheid, C. A., Bratzler, D. W., Leas, B., Stone, E. C., Kelz, R. R., et al. Centers for Disease Control and Prevention Guideline for the Prevention of Surgical Site Infection, 2017. *JAMA Surg.*, 2017; 152(8):784 - 791.

[4] Sørensen, L. T. Wound healing and infection in surgery. The clinical impact of smoking and smoking cessation: a systematic review and meta-analysis. *Arch. Surg.*, 2012; 147(4):373 - 83.

[5] Bowater, R. J., Stirling, S. A., Lilford, R. J. Is antibiotic prophylaxis in surgery a generally effective intervention? Testing a generic hypothesis over a set of meta-analyses. *Ann. Surg.*, 2009; 249(4):551 - 556.

[6] Alexander, J. W., Solomkin, J. S., Edwards, M. J., Updated recommendations for control of surgical site infections. *Ann. Surg.*, 2011; 253(6):1082 - 1093.

[7] Liu, Z., Dumville, J. C., Norman, G., Westby, M. J., Blazeby, J., McFarlane, E., et al. Intraoperative interventions for preventing surgical site infection: an overview of Cochrane Reviews. *Cochrane Database of Systematic Reviews*, 2018, Issue 2. Art. No.: CD012653. DOI: 10.1002/14651858.CD012653.pub2.

[8] Ruiz Tovar, J., Badia, J. M. Prevention of surgical site infection in abdominal surgery. A critical review of the evidence. *Cir. Esp.*, 2014; 92(4):223 - 231.

[9] de Jonge, S. W., Gans, S. L., Atema, J. J., Solomkin, J. S., Dellinger, P. E., Boermeester, M. A. Timing of preoperative antibiotic prophylaxis in 54,552 patients and the risk of surgical site infection: A systematic review and meta-analysis. *Medicine*, (Baltimore) [Internet] 2017; 96. Available at: https://www.ncbi.nlm.nih.gov/pmc/articles/PMC5521876/pdf/medi-96-e6903.pdf.

[10] Kirby, A., Asín-Prieto, E., Burns, F. A., Ewin, D., Fatania, K., Kailavasan, M., et al. Colo-Pro: a pilot randomised controlled trial to compare standard bolus-dosed cefuroxime prophylaxis to bolus-continuous infusion-dosed cefuroxime prophylaxis for the prevention of infections after colorectal surgery. *Eur. J. Clin. Microbiol. Infect. Dis.*, 2019; 38(2):357 - 363.

[11] Peppard, W. J., Eberle, D. G., Kugler, N. W., Mabrey, D. M., Weigelt, J. A., Association between Pre-Operative Cefazolin Dose and Surgical Site Infection in Obese Patients. *Surg. Infect.*, (Larchmt). 2017; 18(4):485 – 490.

[12] Hussain, Z., Curtain, C., Mirkazemi, C., Gadd, K., Peterson, G. M., Zaidi, S. T. R., Prophylactic Cefazolin Dosing and Surgical Site Infections: Does the Dose Matter in Obese Patients. *Obes. Surg.*, 2019; 29(1):159 - 165.

[13] Zapata-Copete, J., Aguilera-Mosquera, S., García-Perdomo, H. A. Antibiotic prophylaxis in breast reduction surgery: a systematic

review and meta-analysis. *J. Plast. Reconstr. Aesthet. Surg.,* 2017; 70(12):1689 - 1695.

[14] Simons, M. P., Smietanski, M., Bonjer, H. J., Bittner, R., Miserez, M., Aufenacker, T. J., et.al. International guidelines for groin hernia management. *Hernia,* 2018; 22(1):1 - 165.

[15] Vamvakidis, K., Rellos, K., Tsourma, M., Christoforides, C., Anastasiou, E., Zorbas, K. A. et al. Antibiotic prophylaxis for clean neck surgery. *Ann. R Coll. Surg. Engl.,* 2017; 99(5):410 - 412.

[16] Sarkut, P., Kilicturgay, S., Aktas, H., Ozen, Y., Kaya, E. Routine Use of Prophylactic Antibiotics during Laparoscopic Cholecystectomy Does Not Reduce the Risk of Surgical Site Infections. *Surg. Infect.,* (Larchmt). 2017; 18(5):603 – 609.

[17] Matsui, Y., Satoi, S., Kaibori, M., Toyokawa, H., Yanagimoto, H., Matsui, K., et al. Antibiotic prophylaxis in laparoscopic cholecystectomy: a randomized controlled trial. *PloS One,* [Internet] 2014; 9. Available at: https://www.ncbi.nlm.nih.gov/pmc/articles/ PMC4156368/pdf/pone.0106702.pdf.

[18] Matsui, Y., Satoi, S., Hirooka, S., Kosaka, H., Kawaura, T., Kitawaki, T., Reappraisal of previously reported meta-analyses on antibiotic prophylaxis for low-risk laparoscopic cholecystectomy: an overview of systematic reviews. *BMJ Open,* [Internet] 2018; 8. Available at: https://www.ncbi.nlm.nih.gov/pmc/articles/ PMC585 7705/pdf/bmjopen-2017-016666.pdf.

[19] Ruangsin, S., Laohawiriyakamol, S., Sunpaweravong, S., Mahattanobon, S. The efficacy of cefazolin in reducing surgical site infection in laparoscopic cholecystectomy: a prospective randomized double-blind controlled trial. *Surg. Endosc.,* 2015; 29(4):874 - 881.

In: Prophylaxis of Surgical Site Infection … ISBN: 978-1-53615-615-7
Editors: Jaime Ruiz-Tovar et al. © 2019 Nova Science Publishers, Inc.

Chapter 6

HANDS AND SKIN PREPARATION

Lorena Rodríguez Cazalla,[*] MD, and Cristina Bernabeu Herraiz, MD

Department of General and Digestive Surgery,
University Hospital San Juan, Alicante, Spain

ABSTRACT

Surgical site infection is one of the most frequent complications in abdominal surgery. Hands hygiene and surgical site skin preparation are measures to prevent it. The common techniques are hand scrubbing and hand rubbing, but there is no firm evidence that one type is better than another. Skin preparation is a standard of care that must always be carried out before any invasive procedure and should include an alcohol-based antiseptic agent.

Keywords: surgical site infection, prevention, surgical hand antisepsis, hand hygiene, surgical skin preparation, antiseptic

---

[*] Corresponding Author's Email: lorena.rc2605@gmail.com.

INTRODUCTION

Surgical site infection (SSI) is one of the most frequent complications in abdominal surgery. It represents one of the most important clinical and economic problems for healthcare systems. This complication is associated with longer hospital stay, the decrease in patient's quality of life and the increase in morbidity, mortality and health costs. Currently, SSI represents in the United States of America around 22% of nosocomial infections [1, 2].

There are many different points in the care pathway where prevention of SSI can take place. This includes antiseptic cleansing of the hands for those who are operating on the patient and also the preparation of the patient's skin. This chapter focuses on these two procedures.

SURGICAL HAND PREPARATION

Historically, hands hygiene has been considered a measure of personal care. However, the relationship between hand washing and the spread of the disease was established in the 19th century thanks to the studies of *Semmelweis* in Vienna and *Holmes* in Boston, who established that hospital-acquired infections are transmitted through the hands of health personnel [3]. Currently, hands hygiene is considered one of the most important measures to prevent the spread of pathogens in healthcare settings [4].

The objective of the surgical hand preparation is to decrease the release of skin bacteria from the hands of the surgical team and to avoid contamination of the surgical field, especially in the case of unnoticed rupture of the sterile glove during the procedure, since the surgical glove is the most important barrier for the migration of microorganisms between the hands of the surgical team and the patient [5, 6]. However, 18% (range: 5-82%) of sterile gloves present perforations after surgery, and over 80% of the cases these perforations are unnoticed by the surgeon. After two hours of surgery, 35% of sterile gloves showed puncture [7].

Surgical hand antisepsis is perhaps the oldest preventative measure used to decrease the incidence of SSI and whose technique has changed most in recent years; for example, during the 19th and 20th century the friction of the skin with a brush was very important but nowadays this practice is totally discouraged due to the skin damages that produces (it is recommended that the friction will be done with the palm of the hand or with a soapy sponge for a single use) [8].

Leclair in 1990 defined antiseptic as "a chemical agent that reduces the microbial population on the skin" [9]. The ideal antiseptic is one that significantly decreases the number of microorganisms in contact with the skin, has broad spectrum, acts quickly with lasting effect, does not produce skin irritation or toxicity and its repeated use is safe [10]. At present, there are several available antiseptic agents, such as:

- Alcohols (60-95%): broad spectrum, fast speed of action, no persistent activity, flammable.
- Chlorhexidine (0.5-4%): broad spectrum, intermediate speed of action, persistent activity, good tolerability, may damage inner ear, eyes and nerve tissue.
- Iodophors (0.5-10%): broad spectrum, intermediate speed of action, decreased effectiveness on contact with organic material, skin irritant, contraindicated in pregnant women, babies and during lactation.
- Phenol derivates (0.5-4%): slow speed of action, no persistent activity, activity neutralized by non-ionic surfactants.
- Triclosan (0.1-2%): no action against viruses and fungi, intermediate speed of action, persistent activity.

Surgical Hand Scrubbing

Surgical hand scrubbing is defined by antisepsis with water and aqueous solution. The most common solutions used for surgical hand scrubbing are chlorhexidine gluconate and povidone iodine.

The application technique, according to World Health Association (WHO), consists of: 1. Scrub each side of each finger, between the fingers, and the back and front of the hand for 2 minutes; 2. Scrub the arms, keeping the hand higher than the arm for all time, wash each side of the arm from the wrist to the elbow for 1 minute; 3. Repeat the process on the other hand and arm; 4. Rinse hands and arms by passing them through the water from fingertips to elbow; 5. Dry hands and arms with sterile towel [12].

Surgical Hand Rubbing

Surgical hand rubbing is defined by antisepsis with alcohol-based solutions, also called waterless scrub.

The application technique, according to the WHO, has a duration of 2 minutes and consists of: 1. Apply 5 ml of solution in the palm of the left hand; 2. Introduce the fingers of the right hand into the solution; 3. Extend the rest of the solution by the right hand upwards reaching the elbow; 4. Apply 5 ml of solution on the right palm and repeat steps 2, 3 and 4 with the left hand and arm; 5. Apply 5 ml more on the left palm by rubbing the solution between the fingers of both hands until the wrists [12].

Recommendations

The Association for Perioperative Practice (AfPP 2011) recommends a prewash with soap and water prior to the first antisepsis of the day to remove dirt (organic material). Most guidelines forbid the use of jewelry, watches or artificial nails in the surgical team's hands [13].

In 2016, Tanner et al. performed a review of four studies about the effect of hand antisepsis in the prevention of SSI and they concluded that there is no strong evidence about the best hand antisepsis. It seems that chlorhexidine reduces the bacterial load on hands more than povidone iodine, but less than the compounds combined with alcohol [9].

Benedetta et al., reviewed six studies (three randomized clinical trials and three observational studies) that compared hand rubbing with hand scrubbing without significant differences related to the incidence of SSI [14].

The WHO recommends that surgical hand preparation be done either by scrubbing with a suitable antimicrobial soap and water or using an alcohol-based hand rub before donning sterile gloves (*strong recommendation, moderate quality of evidence*) [14].

SURGICAL SKIN PREPARATION

The goal of surgical site skin preparation with antiseptics is to reduce the microbial load of the skin before incision and, therefore, decreasing the incidence of SSI [14]. Decontamination of the skin is a standard of care that must always be carried out before any invasive procedure [15, 16].

The three agents mostly used in the surgical site skin preparation are chlorhexidine gluconate, povidone iodine and alcohols, although there are many more available options [4, 15].

The alcoholic compounds are the most microbiologically active agents, but its anti-microbial effect disappears after a few minutes, are inflammable and contraindicated on mucose membranes. Its use for surgical preparation has therefore been practically discontinued. Antiseptics such as chlorhexidine gluconate and povidone iodine are less active than alcohol, but have a greater residual effect. Both can be found in aqueous or alcoholic solutions, the latter being more effective [17].

There are several randomized clinical trials that have compared chlorhexidine-based antiseptics with iodine-based antiseptics in the preoperative preparation of the skin. Most of them have been underpowered to detect differences in SSI rates [18]. Benedetta et al. performed a meta-analysis of twelve randomized clinical trials and they concluded that alcohol-based antiseptics solutions were more effective than aqueous solutions in reducing the risk of SSI (combined OR 0.60 [0.45-0.78]). More specifically, a decrease in SSI risk was observed when comparing the use of alcoholic chlorhexidine with aqueous povidone iodine (combined OR 0.65 [0.47-0.90]) [14]. However, it is important to bear in mind that these studies are comparing two antiseptics combined (chlorhexidine and alcohol) against just one (povidone iodine), attributing the disinfecting power to chlorhexidine and forgetting the role of alcohol [19]. A recent clinical trial showed that the use of alcoholic chlorhexidine for preoperative skin antisepsis at cesarean delivery was associated with a significantly lower risk of SSI than was the use of iodine–alcohol [20].

The recommendations of the main scientific societies are:

- *NICE (2013):* prepare the skin at the surgical site immediately before incision using an antiseptic (aqueous or alcohol-based) preparation, povidone-iodine or chlorhexidine are most suitable [21].
- *Cochrane (2015):* preoperative skin preparation with 0.5% chlorhexidine in methylated spirits was associated with lower rates of SSIs following clean surgery than alcohol-based povidone iodine [10].
- *WHO (2016):* the panel recommends alcohol-based antiseptic solutions that are based on chlorhexidine gluconate for surgical site skin preparation (*strong recommendation; low to moderate quality of evidence*) [14].
- *CDC (2017):* perform skin preparation with an alcohol-based antiseptic agent unless contraindicated (*strong recommendation; high-quality evidence*) [22].

The antiseptic agent must be applied with a specific applicator or sterile capsule, clamp and gauze, brushing the skin with forward and backward movements. The application must be carried out for about 30 seconds, allowing the product to dry for at least 2 minutes [23].

REFERENCES

[1] Anthony T, Long T, Hynan LS, Sarosi GAJ, Nwariaku F, Huth J, et al. Surgical complications exert a lasting effect on disease-specific health-related quality of life for patients with colorectal cancer. *Surgery.* 2003;134(2):119-125.

[2] Magill S, Edwards J, Bamberg W, Beldavs Z, Dumyati G, Kainer M, et al. Multitaste point-prevalence survey of health care-associated infections. *N Engl J Med.* 2014;370(13):1198-1208.

[3] Best M, Neuhauser D. Ignaz Semmelweis and the birth of infection control. *Qual Saf Health Care.* 2004;13(3):233-234.

[4] Boyce JM, Pittet D, Healthcare Infection Control Practices Advisory Committe, HICPAC/SHEA/APICIDSA Hand Hygiene Task Force. Guideline for Hand Hygiene in Health-Care Settings. Recommendations of the Healthcare Infection Control Disease Practices Advisory Committee and the HICPAC/SHEA/APIC/IDSA Hand Hygiene Task Force. Society for Healthcare Epidemiology of America/Association for Professionals in Infection Control/ Infectious Diseases Society of America. *MMWR Recomm Rep.* 2002;51(RR-16):1-45.

[5] Kampf G, Goroncy-Bermes P, Fraise A, Rotter M. Terminology in surgical hand desinfection- a new Tower of Babel in infection control. *J Hosp Infect.* 2005;59(3):269-271.

[6] Hübner NO, Goerdt AM, Stanislawski N, Assadian O, Heidecke CD, Kramer A, et al. Bacterial migration through punctured surgical gloves under real surgical conditions. *BMC Infect Dis* [Internet] 2010;10. Available at: https://www.ncbi.nlm.nih.gov/pmc/articles/PMC2909237/pdf/1471-2334-10-192.pdf.

[7] Widmer A. Surgical hand hygiene: scrub or rub?. *J Hosp Infect.* 2013;83 (Suppl 1):S35-S39.

[8] Widmer A, Rotter M, Voss A, Nthumba P, Allegranzi B, Boyce J, et al. Surgical hand preparation: state-of-the-art. *J Hosp Infect.* 2010;74(2):112-122.

[9] Tanner J, Dumville J, Norman G, Fortnam M. Surgical hand antisepsis to reduce surgical site infection. *Cochrane Database of Systematic Reviews 2016,* Issue 1. Art. No.: CD004288. DOI: 10.1002/14651858.CD004288.pub3.

[10] Dumville JC, McFarlane E, Edwards P, Lipp A, Holmes A, Liu Z. Preoperative skin antiseptics for preventing surgical wound infections after clean surgery. *Cochrane Database of Systematic Reviews* 2015, Issue 4. Art. No.: CD003949. DOI: 10.1002/14651858.CD003949.pub4.

[11] Machet L, Fourtillan E, Vaillant L. Antisépticos. *EMC Tratado de Medicina.* Elsevier; 2016.

[12] World Health Organization. Surgical hand preparation: state-of-the-art. In *WHO Guidelines on Hand Hygiene in Health Care: First Global Patient Safety Challenge Clean Care is Safer Care.* Geneva; World Health Organization; 2009. p. 54-60.

[13] *The Association for Perioperative Practice* [Internet]. United Kingdom; 2011. Available at: http://afpp.org.uk/books-journal/books/book-123.

[14] Allegranzi B, Bischoff P, De Jonge S, Kubilay NZ, Zayed B, Gomes SM, et al. New WHO recommendations on preoperative measures for surgical site infection prevention: an evidence-based global perspective. *Lancet Infect Dis.* 2016;16(12):e276-e287.

[15] Sidhwa F, Itani K. Skin preparation before surgery: Options and Evidence. *Surg Infect (Larchmt).* 2015;16(1):14-23.

[16] Anderson DJ, Podgorny K, Berríos-Torres SI, Bratzler DW, Dellinger EP, Greene L, et al. Strategies to prevent surgical site infections in acute care hospitals: 2014 update. *Infect Control Hosp Epidemiol.* 2014;35(6):605-627.

[17] Ruíz-Tovar J, Badia JM. Prevention of surgical site infection in abdominal surgery. A critical review of the evidence. *Cir Esp.* 2014;92(4):223-231.

[18] Ban KA, Minei JP, Laronga C, Harbrecht BG, Jensen EH, Fry DE, et al. American College of Surgeons and Surgical Infection Society:

Surgical Site Infection Guidlines, 2016 Update. *J Am Coll Surg.* 2017;224(1):59-74.

[19] Maiwald M, Chan E. The forgotten role of alcohol: a systematic review and meta-analysis of the clinical efficacy and perceived role of chlorhexidine in skin antisepsis. *PLoS One* [Internet] 2007;7. Available at: https://www.ncbi.nlm.nih.gov/pmc/articles/PMC3434203/pdf/pone.0044277.pdf.

[20] Tuuli MG, Liu J, Stout MJ, Martin S, Cahill AG, Odibo AO, et al. A Randomized Trial Comparing Skin Antiseptic Agents at Cesarean Delivery. *N Engl J Med.* 2016;374(7):647-655.

[21] *National Institute for Health and Care Excellence* [Internet]. Available at: http://www.nice.org.uk/guidance/qs49.

[22] Berríos-Torres SI, Umscheid CA, Bratzler DW, Leas B, Stone EC, Kelz RR, et al. Centers for Disease Control and Prevention Guideline for the Prevention of Surgical Site Infection. *JAMA Surg.* 2017;152(8):784-791.

[23] Spanish Society of Preventive Medicine, Public Health and Hygiene. "*Zero Surgical Site Infection*" Project [Internet]; 2017. Available at: http://infeccionquirurgicazero.es/images/stories/recursos/protocolo/2017/3-1-17-documento-Protocolo-IQZ.pdf.

In: Prophylaxis of Surgical Site Infection … ISBN: 978-1-53615-615-7
Editors: Jaime Ruiz-Tovar et al. © 2019 Nova Science Publishers, Inc.

Chapter 7

HYPEROXYGENATION, HYPOTHERMIA PREVENTION, NORMOGLYCEMIA AND NORMOVOLEMIA

Esther García Villabona[*], *MD*
and Carmen Vallejo Lantero, MD
Anesthesiology Department,
Hospital Universitario de La Princesa, Madrid, Spain

ABSTRACT

Surgical site infections (SSIs) are defined as infections anatomically associated with a surgical procedure performed in an operating room and not present prior to the operation. They have been shown to account for up to 16% of healthcare-associated infections. The rate of surgical site infection varies depending on the type of procedure, with rates of less than 1% for orthopaedic procedures and rates of over 10% for large bowel surgery. They can often be prevented with appropriate care before, during and after surgery. [1]

---

[*] Corresponding Author's Email: esthergarciavillabona@gmail.com.

Keywords: surgical site infection, oxygenation, temperature, normovolemia, hiperglycemia.

INTRODUCTION

Surgical site infection (SSI) is a type of healthcare-associated infection in which a surgical incision site becomes infected after a surgical procedure. These infections represent an important problem for patients and a significant financial burden for the health care system. [2]

Many factors in the patient's journey through surgery have been identified as contributing to the risk of SSI. Therefore, the prevention of these infections is complex and requires the integration of a range of preventive measures before, during and after surgery.

There is evidence that optimizing blood flow to the surgical incision, we can decrease surgical site infection rates through the avoidance of hypothermia, hypoxia and decreased perfusion. If an infection does develop, appropriate treatment will minimise morbidity resulting from the infection.

Ideally, perioperative fluid therapy prevents tissue hypoxia by maximizing the cardiac output and thus improving arterial oxygenation. Nevertheless, an adequate assessment of normovolemia remains complicated.

On the other hand, several observational studies showed that hyperglycaemia is associated with an increased risk of SSI in both diabetic and non-diabetic patients. Conflicting results have been reported about the optimal target levels of blood glucose and the ideal timing for glucose control (intra- and/or postoperative).

METHODS

Hyperoxygenation

It has been claimed that patients undergoing surgery with general anesthesia could benefit from a higher than normal inspired oxygen fraction (FiO2). Some authors have suggested that a high FiO2 is a simple, inexpensive, and low risk intervention, and that the broader use of this technique should be encouraged in patients undergoing major abdominal procedures. [3]

Several trials have been published on the use of high fractions of inspired oxygen concentration (FiO2) during the perioperative period and the potential association with lower rates of SSI. This intervention consists of providing patients with 80% oxygen compared to the usual administration of 30% oxygen. Patients are routinely given 100% oxygen for 30 seconds to 2 minutes prior to intubation and then maintained on either "normoxia," defined as oxygen at FiO2 30% or 35%, or "hyperoxia," defined as oxygen at FiO2 80%.

The arguments for providing oxygen levels beyond the standard 30% are largely based on two notions. The first is that the surgical incision may not be adequately perfused and might receive substantially higher oxygen if there is a higher partial pressure of oxygen in the blood. The other concept is that host defense systems might be further improved by higher oxygen partial pressures, particularly by enhancing neutrophil oxidative killing. This argument devolves down to the affinity of the nicotinamide adenine dinucleotide phosphate (NADPH) oxidase for oxygen. The Michaelis constant for the enzyme for oxygen is 5-20 µM Hg O2. It has been shown that oxygen tension at infected sites is greatly reduced compared with most uninfected tissues (PO2 approximating 25 mM of oxygen ≈3% oxygen). [1]

Overall, it has been shown (with a moderate quality of evidence) that increased perioperative FiO2 (80%) is beneficial in reducing SSI when compared to standard perioperative FiO2 (30-35%) in patients undergoing surgical procedures under general anaesthesia with endotracheal intubation. The benefit of hyperoxygenation tended to be greater in open colorectal surgery than in other types of abdominal surgery. Many authors have considered that subgroup as the most likely to profit from a high FiO2. The question then is, whether this benefit is of clinical relevance. Although the degree of antiinfective efficacy of high FiO2 seems weak and perhaps disappointing, it seems to be similar to conventional antibiotic prophylaxis in many surgical settings. As most patients in these trials had received prophylactic antibiotics, we may conclude on the efficacy of high FiO2 as a supplemental antiinfection strategy only. It would be difficult to test the efficacy of high FiO2 alone from an ethical perspective because the administration of prophylactic antibiotics is widely considered as a standard of care. [3]

Potential Harms

Some authors are cautious about the use of increased FiO2. Skepticism has been partly related to the fact that high FiO2 may have deleterious effects on the airways. One hundred percent oxygen at induction or at the end of general anesthesia has been suggested to promote atelectasis over a few minutes, and to cause alteration in gas exchange.

However, this increase in atelectasis has been described after the administration of 100% FiO2 compared to 80% FiO2 and showed a meaningful difference between the two concentrations. Moreover, none of the clinical trials investigating the administration of 80% FiO2 that reported adverse events showed a significant difference in pulmonary complications or other adverse events.

Patients with chronic obstructive pulmonary disease should be evaluated preoperatively and their perioperative anesthesia needs to be designed to minimize complications as the risks of high inspiratory concentrations of oxygen may outweigh the benefits for these patients. [3]

Hypothermia Prevention

Hypothermia is defined as a core temperature below 36°C and is common during and after major surgical procedures lasting more than 2 hours. The human body has a central compartment comprising the major organs where temperature is tightly regulated, and a peripheral compartment where temperature varies widely. Heat loss is compensated by reducing blood flow through the skin and increasing heat production, mainly by inducing muscular activity (shivering) and increasing the basal metabolic rate. Typically, the periphery compartment may be 2°C to 4°C cooler than the core compartment. [4]

Causes of Hypothermia

The most common events leading to hypothermia are the exposure to a cold operating room environment and the anaesthetic-induced impairment of thermoregulatory control.

- Skin surface exposure during the perioperative period can increase heat loss. In addition, cool intravenous and irrigation fluids directly cool patients.
- Sedatives and anaesthetic agents inhibit the normal response to cold, resulting in an improved blood flow to the periphery and increased heat loss.

During the early period of anaesthesia, these effects are seen as a rapid decrease in core temperature caused by redistribution of heat from the central to the peripheral compartment. This early decrease is followed by a more gradual decline, reflecting ongoing heat loss. With epidural or spinal analgesia, the peripheral blockade of vasoconstriction below the level of the nerve block results in vasodilatation and greater ongoing heat loss.

Complications of Hypothermia

Inadvertent non-therapeutic hypothermia is considered to be an adverse effect of general and regional anaesthesia and can cause different complications.

a) Cardiac complications are the principal cause of morbidity during the postoperative phase because of the release of noradrenaline causing peripheral vasoconstriction and hypertension.
b) Prolonged recovery from anaesthesia and a longer length of hospital stay.
c) Even moderate hypothermia (35°C) can alter physiological coagulation mechanisms by affecting platelet function and modifying enzymatic reactions. Decreased platelet activity results in increased bleeding and a greater need for transfusion.
d) Moderate hypothermia can also reduce the metabolic rate, manifesting as a prolonged effect of certain drugs used during anaesthesia and some uncertainty about their effects. This is particularly significant for elderly patients.
e) The maintenance of normothermia might reduce the incidence of surgical site infection, but all available studies in this field measure core and not peripheral temperature. The reported lower core temperatures result in a reduced cutaneous temperature at the operative site. Recent health care bundles and guidelines for SSI prevention recommend that body temperature should be maintained above 35.5-36°C during the perioperative period. [1]

Recommended Measures to Prevent Hypothermia

1. Perioperative care:

   - Patients, relatives and carers should be informed that staying warm before surgery will lower the risk of postoperative complications.
   - When using any temperature recording or warming device, healthcare professionals should be trained in their use.

- Measure the patient's temperature using a site that produces either: a direct measurement of core temperature, or a direct estimate of core temperature that has been shown in research studies to be accurate to within 0.5°C of direct measurement. These sites are: pulmonary artery catheter, distal oesophagus, urinary bladder, zero heat-flux (deep forehead), sublingual, axilla, rectum.

2. Preoperative phase:

The preoperative phase is defined as the hour before induction of anaesthesia, during which the patient is prepared for surgery.

- Each patient should be assessed for their risk of inadvertent perioperative hypothermia and potential adverse consequences before transfer to the theatre suite.
- Patients should be managed as higher risk if any 2 of the following apply:
  a) American Society of Anesthesiologists (ASA) grade II to V (the higher the grade, the greater the risk)
  b) Preoperative temperature below 36.0°C (and preoperative warming is not possible because of clinical urgency)
  c) Undergoing combined general and regional anaesthesia
  d) Undergoing major or intermediate surgery
  e) At risk of cardiovascular complications
- The patient's temperature should be measured and documented in the hour before the surgery.
- If the patient's temperature is below 36.0°C, start active warming preoperatively unless there is a need to expedite surgery because of clinical urgency.
- If the patient's temperature is 36.0°C or above, start active warming at least 30 minutes before induction of anaesthesia, unless this will delay emergency surgery.

- Forced air warming seems to have beneficial effect in terms of a lower rate of surgical site infection and complications, at least in those undergoing abdominal surgery, compared to not applying any active warming systems.
- Maintain active warming throughout the intraoperative phase.
- On transfer to the theatre suite:
  - active warming should be continued (or re-started as soon as possible)
  - the patient should be encouraged to walk to theatre where appropriate.

3. Intraoperative phase

The intraoperative phase is defined as total anaesthesia time, from the first anaesthetic intervention through to patient transfer to the recovery area of the theatre suite.

- The patient's temperature should be measured and documented before induction of anaesthesia and then every 30 minutes until the end of surgery.
- Induction of anaesthesia should not begin unless the patient's temperature is 36.0°C or above (unless there is a need to expedite surgery because of clinical urgency, for example bleeding or critical limb ischaemia).
- In the theatre suite the ambient temperature should be at least 21°C while the patient is exposed. The ambient temperature may be reduced once active warming is established to allow better working conditions using equipment to cool the surgical team.
- The patient should be adequately covered throughout the intraoperative phase to conserve heat, and exposed only during surgical preparation.
- Intravenous fluids (500 ml or more) and blood products should be warmed to 37°C using a fluid warming device.

- Warm patients intraoperatively from induction of anaesthesia, using a forced-air warming device, if they are:
  a) having anaesthesia for more than 30 minutes or
  b) having anaesthesia for less than 30 minutes and are at higher risk of inadvertent perioperative hypothermia.

Consider a resistive heating mattress or resistive heating blanket if a forced-air warming device is unsuitable.

- The temperature setting on forced-air warming devices should be set at maximum and then adjusted to maintain a patient temperature of at least 36.5°C.
- All irrigation fluids used intraoperatively should be warmed in a thermostatically controlled cabinet to a temperature of 38°C to 40°C.

4. Postoperative phase

The postoperative phase is defined as the 24 hours after the patient has entered the recovery area of the theatre suite.

- The patient's temperature should be measured and documented on admission to the recovery room and then every 15 minutes.
- If the patient's temperature is below 36.0°C, they should be actively warmed using forced-air warming until they are discharged from the recovery room or until they are comfortably warm.
- Patients should be kept comfortably warm when back on the ward.
- If the patient's temperature falls below 36.0°C while on the ward: they should be warmed using forced-air warming until they are comfortably warm. Their temperature should be measured and documented at least every 30 minutes during warming [4, 5].

Hyperglycemia Prevention

Blood glucose levels rise during and after surgery due to surgical stress. Surgery causes a stress response that results in a release of catabolic hormones and the inhibition of insulin. Moreover, surgical stress influences pancreatic beta-cell function, which results in lower plasma insulin levels. Taken together, this relative hypoinsulinaemia, insulin resistance and excessive catabolism from the action of counter-regulatory hormones make surgical patients at high risk for hyperglycaemia, even non-diabetic patients. [6]

Several observational studies showed that hyperglycaemia is associated with an increased risk of SSI and therefore an increased risk of morbidity, mortality and higher health care costs in both diabetic and non-diabetic patients and in different types of surgery .

A recent systematic review and cohort meta-analysis including 16 studies [7] concluded that use of an evidence- based, surgical care bundle for patients undergoing colorectal surgery significantly reduced the risk of SSI. Although none of the studies in this analysis used the identical SSI care bundles, all included elements from a core group of interventions, including appropriate antibiotic prophylaxis, normothermia, appropriate hair removal, and glycemic control for hyperglycemic patients.

Hyperglycemia is a known risk factor for infection because it impedes the normal physiologic responses to infection. In vivo studies show that hyperglycemia is associated with accelerated nonenzymatic glycosylation of proteins or the nonenzymatic addition of sugar molecules to the exposed lysine residues on extracellular proteins. Short-term glycosylation of immunoglobulins inactivates them. Furthermore, hyperglycemia impairs leukocyte function, including abnormalities in granulocyte adherence, impaired phagocytosis, delayed chemotaxis, and depressed bactericidal activity. The degree of hyperglycemia that has been shown to impair phagocytic function, both in vivo and in vitro, is approximately 200 mg/dL. More important, the degree of phagocytic impairment can be reversed with control of glucose level. [8]

Conflicting results have been reported regarding the different treatment options to control hyperglycaemia in diabetic and non- diabetic patients, the optimal target levels of blood glucose and the ideal timing for glucose control (intra- and/or postoperative). The general consensus remains that glucose levels greater than 200 mg/dL is detrimental, but the lower limit and the tightness of control is debatable. Moreover, some studies targeting relatively low perioperative glucose levels have highlighted the risk of adverse effects associated with intensive protocols as they may cause hypoglycaemia. [9]

Overall low-quality evidence shows that a protocol with more strict blood glucose target levels has a significant benefit in reducing SSI rates when compared to a conventional protocol. There was evidence that the effect was smaller in studies that used intensive blood glucose controls intraoperatively only compared to studies that used an intensive protocol postoperatively or both intra- and postoperatively.

Meta-regression analysis showed that the benefit of an intensive protocol over a conventional protocol was consistent in both patients with and those without diabetes, and whether commenced during or after surgery. Among the intensive protocols, the effect was similar in studies with a target blood glucose level of ≤110 mg/dL and an upper limit target level of 110-150 mg/dL. [10]

Five studies reported significantly more hypoglycaemic measurements in the intensive group compared with the control group. Although these events were asymptomatic, with none of the studies reporting clinical consequences, it remains unknown to what extent these hypoglycaemic episodes harm patients in the long term and whether this potential harm outweighs the reduced risk of SSI. [10]

Targeting stricter and lower blood glucose levels with an intensive protocol of perioperative glucose control reduces SSI without increasing the risk of death or stroke. Although the optimal target level cannot be derived from published data, the summary data of present systematic review and meta-analysis indicate that target glucose levels of less than 150 mg/dl in the perioperative period can be achieved safely with minimal risk of asymptomatic hypoglycaemic events and with no significant increase in serious adverse events. [10]

Due to the risk of hypoglycaemia, targeting lower levels should be avoided. While most recommendations focus on the diabetic patient only, those issuedby SHEA/IDSA and the American College of Physicians apply to all surgical patients. They recommend either target levels between 140-200 mg/dL or upper limits of 180 mg/dL or 198 mg/dL. [6]

Thus, the Global Guidelines for the prevention of surgical site infection endorsed by WHO, unanimously agreed that the recommendation to use protocols for intensive perioperative blood glucose control should apply to both diabetics and non-diabetics. However, the available evidence did not allow the definition of an optimal target level of blood glucose. [6]

Normovolemia

Wound infections are serious complications of surgery. Oxidative killing by neutrophils is the most important defense against pathogens causing surgical infections. Because oxygen is the substrate for oxidative killing, the rate of bacterial killing depends on sufcient tissue oxygenation. Wound healing and resistance to infection are dependent on tissue oxygen tension. Sufficient tissue oxygenation is essential for collagen synthesis and wound repair and is improved by adequate arterial oxygenation. [11]Ideally, perioperative fluid therapy prevents tissue hypoxia by maximizing the cardiac output and thus improving arterial oxygenation.

Fluid overload leads to a decrease in muscular oxygen tension. Due to surgical trauma, a systemic inflammatory response arises, which leads to a fluid shift to the extravascular space. Following a large fluid shift, generalized oedema may occur, which decreases tissue oxygenation and impedes tissue healing. By contrast, hypovolemia leads to arterial and tissue hypoxia due to a decrease in cardiac output. The optimal fluid (colloid or crystalloid) or strategy of fluid management (goal-directed, liberal or restricted) remains a subjet of controversy. [1]

Perioperative goal-directed therapy (GDT) aims to match the increased oxygen demand incurred during major surgery, by flow-based haemodynamic monitoring and therapeutic interventions to achieve a predetermined haemodynamic endpoint. [12] Several metaanalyses of RCTs have shown that goal-directed fluid therapy (GDT) reduces postoperative morbidity and length of hospital stay, especially in high-risk patients undergoing major surgery.

Few organizations have issued recommendations regarding the maintenance of normovolemia. The UK-based NICE recommends maintaining adequate perfusion during surgery. Based on an evidence update in 2013, it is stated that haemodynamic GDT appears to reduce SSI rates. [6]

Overall low quality evidence shows that intraoperative GDT has significant benefit in reducing the SSI rate compared to standard fluid management. This effect is shown also for GDT in the postoperative period. Considering the low quality evidence above-mentioned, the WHO in the second edition of the Global Guidelines for the prevention of surgical site infection agreed to suggest the use of GDT intraoperatively and decided that the strength of this recommendation should be conditional. [6] The guidelines developers group highlighted that a widely-accepted definition for normovolemia is needed. Future studies including large well-designed RCTs with clear definitions should aim at identifying the most accurate and least invasive method of measuring normovolemia and assess its influence with regard to tissue oxygenation and normothermia.

Peri-operative goal-directed therapy, using fluids and/or inotropes, typically involves the use of haemodynamic targets to optimize oxygen delivery. A systematic literature search identified three haemodynamic management goals: stroke volume optimization by fluid therapy; maintenance of a target mean arterial pressure by vasopressor therapy; maintenance of a target cardiac index ≥ 2.5 l/min per m^2 by inotropic therapy. [13] The use of an algorithm is helpful, while considering that local resources and expertise may vary and limit possibilities for the optimal strategy. Indeed, the variety of effective algorithms on a multitude of outcomes indicates that having an algorithm for a specific goal is the most important factor, more than any particular algorithm associated with the effect of GDT.

CONCLUSION

During surgery patients are kept in a stable condition by the operating team. All tissues heal most effectively in optimal conditions of oxygenation, perfusion and body temperature.

Intraoperative high FiO2 may be regarded as a supplemental strategy to further decrease the risk of surgical site infection in patients receiving prophylactic antibiotics without increasing the risk of postoperative atelectasis.

Inadvertent perioperative hypothermia is a common but preventable complication of perioperative procedures that is associated with an increased risk of surgical site infection and other postoperative complications. Surgical patients are at risk of developing hypothermia before, during or after surgery. Maintaining normothermia throughout this period (except if cooling is required for medical reasons) will therefore reduce the risk of infection at the surgical site and ensure that patients feel comfortably warm at all times.

Hyperglycemia is a known risk factor for infection. Overall low-quality evidence shows that a protocol of control for blood glucose levels has a significant benefit in reducing SSI rates. The effect was similar in studies with a more intensive target blood glucose level and an upper limit target. Available evidence did not allow the definition of an optimal target level of blood glucose. Due to the risk of hypoglycaemia, targeting lower levels should be avoided.

At present, there is no universal definition of normovolemia or a standardized method for its assessment. Low quality evidence shows that intraoperative GDT has significant benefit in reducing the SSI rate. Considering that both fluid overload and hypovolemia are likely to affect other clinical outcomes, actual recommendations suggest the use of GDT intraoperatively, but the strength of this recommendation should be conditional.

REFERENCES

[1] World Health Organization. *Global guidelines for the prevention of surgical site infection.* WHO, Geneva; 2016.

[2] National Institute for Health and Care Excellence. Surgical site infection: prevention and treatment of surgical site infection. *Clinical guideline 74*. NICE, London 2008. Last updated: February 2017.

[3] Hovaguimian F, Lysakowski C, Elia N, Tramèr MR; Effect of intraoperative high inspired oxygen fraction on surgical site infection, postoperative nausea and vomiting, and pulmonary function: systematic review and meta-analysis of randomized controlled trials. *Anesthesiology.* 2013 Aug:119(2):303-16. doi: 10.1097/ALN.0b013e31829aaff4.

[4] National Institute for Health and Care Excellence. Hypothermia: prevention and management in adults having surgery. *Clinical guideline 65*. NICE, London 2008. Last updated: December 2016.

[5] Madrid E, Urrútia G, Roqué I Figuls M, Pardo-Hernández H, Campos JM, Paniagua P, Maestre L, Alonso-Coello P. Active body surface warming systems for preventing complications caused by inadvertent perrioperative hypothermia in adults. *Cochrane Database Syst Rev.* 2016 Apr 21; 4:CD009016. doi: 10.1002/14651858.

[6] *Global guidelines for the prevention of surgical site infection*, second edition ISBN 978-92-4-155047-5. World Health Organization 2018.

[7] Carmichael JC, Keller DS, Baldini G, et al. Clinical Practice Guidelines for Enhanced Recovery After Colon and Rectal Surgery from the American Society of Colon and Rectal Surgeons and Society of American Gastrointestinal and Endoscopic Surgeons. *Dis Colon Rectum* 2017; 60: 761–784.

[8] Ng R, Oo A, Liu W, et al. Changing glucose control target and risk of surgical site infection in a Southeast Asian population. *J Thorac Cardiovasc Surg.* 2015;149(1):323-8.

[9] Griesdale DE, de Souza RJ, van Dam RM, Heyland DK, Cook DJ, Malhotra A, et al. Intensive insulin therapy and mortality among critically ill patients: a meta-analysis including NICE-SUGAR study data. *CMAJ.* 2009;180(8):821-827.

[10] De Vries FEE, Gans SL, Solomkin JS, et al. Meta-analysis of lower perioperative blood glucose target levels for reduction of surgical-site infection. *BJS* 2017; 104: e95–e105.

[11] Kabon B, Akca O, Taguchi A, Nagele A, Jebadurai R, Arkilic CF, et al. Supplemental intravenous crystalloid administration does not reduce the risk of surgical wound infection. *Anesth Analg.* 2005;101:1546-53.

[12] Cecconi M, Corredor C, Arulkumaran N, Abuella G, et al. Clinical review: Goal-directed therapy. What is the evidence in surgical patients? The effect on different risk groups. *Crit Care* 2013;17:209.

[13] Feldheiser A, Conroy P, Bonomo T, et al. Development and feasibility study of an algorithm for intraoperative goal directed haemodynamic management in noncardiac surgery. *J Int Med Res* 2012;40: 1227-1241.

In: Prophylaxis of Surgical Site Infection … ISBN: 978-1-53615-615-7
Editors: Jaime Ruiz-Tovar et al. © 2019 Nova Science Publishers, Inc.

Chapter 8

ADHESIVES AND WOUND PROTECTORS

Dennis César Lévano-Linares[1,][*], MD and Patricia Sanchez-Salcedo[2], RN

[1]Department of Surgery, University Hospital Rey Juan Carlos,
Mostoles, Madrid, Spain
[2]Department of Surgical Nursery, Fundacion Jimenez Diaz,
Madrid, Spain

ABSTRACT

Surgical site infections (SSI) are the most frequent complications in surgery procedures. Despite the use of standard surgical techniques (antiseptic skin preparation, sterile draping, and antibiotics) that could prevent perioperative wound infections, wound infection following clean-contaminated procedures occurs in more than 10%. SSI contribute substantially to postoperative morbidity and mortality and have been shown to significantly increase the mean length of hospital stays and treatment costs. Thus, devices to reduce SSI incidence are of great medical and economic importance. Adhesive draps and plastic wound protectors were originally designed to be a simple, easy-to-use, and cost-effective device that reduces the contact between bacteria and incisions,

---

[*] Corresponding Author's Email: cesdenlinares@gmail.com.

and provides a relatively disease-free environment for the operator, which could reduce the SSI substantially.

Keywords: surgical site infections, plastic wound protectors, wound infection

INTRODUCTION

Surgical site infection (SSI) is one of the most common hospital acquired infections in the field of surgery. SSI leads to increased overall health care cost and is associated with a prolonged hospital stay, more complex wound care needs, more frequent visits to outpatient clinics, and higher rates of hospital readmission and morbidities [1]. Thus, SSI rates have been used to evaluate outcome measures of surgical quality worldwide. Risk factors affecting the SSI rate can be categorized into 2 main groups: patient related and procedure related [2]. Patient-related factors include generally nonmodifiable factors such as patient age, body mass index, malnutrition, comorbidities (such as uncontrolled diabetes mellitus or anemia), and American Society of Anesthesiologists (ASA) score. Meanwhile, procedure-related factors can be controlled to a degree and therefore may be modified in an effort to reduce the risk of SSI; these include the method of skin preparation, meticulous dissection and reduced operating time, use of minimally invasive surgery compared with conventional open surgery, and use of prophylactic antibiotics. Physical wound protection can reduce the rate of SSI in patients undergoing abdominal surgery. Most abdominal surgeries are performed with a clean-contaminated or contaminated-incisional wound because these often require manipulation or resection of the bowel or biliary tract. In particular, emergency abdominal surgeries are more likely to consist of contaminated and dirty wounds. Therefore, in these cases, it is especially important to physically protect the incisional wound from sources of infection such as bowel content spillage to reduce the SSI rate. Adhesive drapes, antimicrobial skin sealants and impervious plastic wound protectors

(IPWP)—so-called wound edge protectors, circular wound edge protectors or plastic ring wound protectors—have been used to protect the incisional wound and reduce SSI rates [3]. However, the effectiveness of these wound protectors on reducing the SSI rate remains unclear. For example, despite the expected clinical benefit of IPWP to reduce the rate of SSIs and the favorable results reported by several studies [4], some prospective series and randomized clinical trials (RCT) have reported disappointing results of the effect of IPWPs on reducing SSI rates in patients undergoing abdominal surgery [5]. In this chapter, we will analyze the effectiveness of each of the devices used in the protection of the skin and the surgical wound in patients undergoing abdominal surgery and the updated recommendations on their use.

WOUND PROTECTORS

The use of adhesive membrane barriers over the skin of the surgical site emerged 50 years ago as a possible solution to minimise endogenous cross-contamination during surgery [6]. The initial idea relied on the principle of reducing exposure of the surgical site to bacteria inherent in the surrounding skin or to airborne bacteria in the operating room. Major applicability was expected in clean surgeries, where the skin is considered the main source of bacteria. Unfortunately, however, no evidence in support of plastic adhesive drapes was found in a recently updated systematic review RCT including five studies and 3082 participants(2). In fact, a 23% increase in the risk of SSI was found in the group that received adhesive drapes. In the 1960s, other devices were described and then developed based on the concept of combining a non-traumatic surgical wound retractor with a protective membrane covering of the incisional margin in abdominal surgeries. Such protective covers or 'wound protectors' were hypothesised to be an improvement over adhesive membrane barriers as they were believed to reduce intraoperative contamination while concomitantly preserving the temperature and humidity of the surgical wound. In support of this hypothesis, early studies demonstrated reduced exposure of the surgical wound to enteric bacteria at the end of gastrointestinal operations [7, 8]. These results were further supported by several RCT, which demonstrated that wound protectors were efficacious in reducing the incidence of incisional SSI as compared to usual care in patients undergoing gastrointestinal surgeries [4, 9, 10]. There are different impervious circular wound edge protectors (CWEP), but they all fall into two main categories: a.) devices with a single semirigid plastic ring placed into the abdominal cavity after laparotomy with an impervious drape attached, which comes out of the abdomen to protect the incisional edges (single-ring device) and b.) devices with two semi-rigid plastic rings connected by an impervious drape (Figure 1).

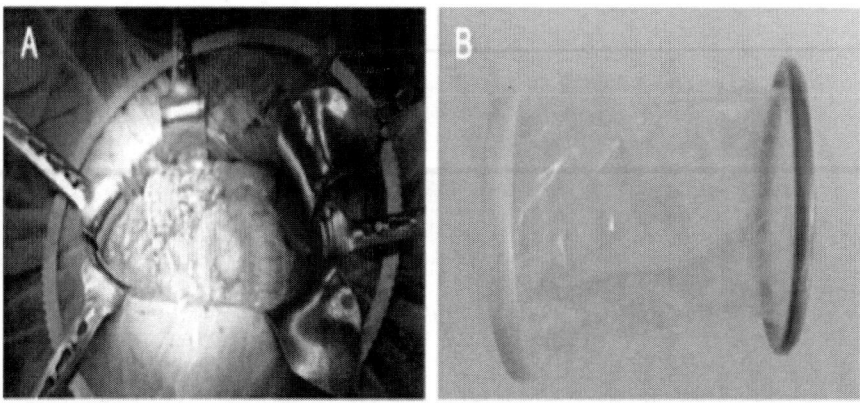

Figure 1. Circular wound edge protectors (CWEP). A single-ring device. B double-ring device [11].

Table 1. Recommendations on the use of WP devices according to available guidelines [14]

Guidelines (year issued)	Recommendations on the use of WP devices
SHEA/IDSA practice recommendation (2014)	Use impervious plastic WPs for gastrointestinal and biliary tract surgery.
NICE (2013 update)	Wound edge protection devices may reduce the SSI rate after open abdominal surgery, but the current lack of high-quality studies implies that more research is needed.

These new surgical devices comprise a non-adhesive plastic sheath attached to a single or double rubber ring that firmly secures the sheath to the wound edges. The device is intended to facilitate the retraction of the incision during surgery without the need for additional mechanical retractors and cloths. Theoretically, commercially-available CWEP are intended to reduce wound edge contamination to a minimum during abdominal surgical procedures, including contamination from outside (clean surgery) and inside the peritoneal cavity (clean-contaminated, contaminated and dirty surgery). Although these surgical devices are already on the market, their real usefulness and cost-effectiveness warrants additional evidence-based analysis. Few organizations have issued recommendations regarding the use of CWEP devices. The UK-based NICE states that wound edge protection devices may reduce SSI rates after open abdominal surgery, but no recommendation is given due to the lack of further high-quality evidence [12]. However, SHEA/IDSA guidelines recommend the use of impervious plastic CWEP for gastrointestinal and biliary tract surgery [13].

While CWEP effectively protect wound edges from bacterial invasion their clinical effectiveness has been disputed and their widespread use has been hampered by conflicting trial results with some authors reporting beneficial effects [10] while others found no benefit [15].

Two previous smaller reviews based on limited patient numbers and low-quality evidence reported a beneficial effect of CWEP, but called for adequately powered, high-quality trials [16] which have been conducted since then. A recently meta-analysis of RCT, evaluated whether diverse types of wound protectors may reduce the risk of SSI among patients undergoing gastrointestinal or biliary surgery [17]. Among six trials, which enrolled 1008 patients, it was found that the pooled estimated risk of SSI among patients fitted with wound protectors during surgery was 0.55 (95% CI 0.31 to 0.98) times the pooled estimated risk of SSI in control groups. Moreover, among patients treated with dual-ring versus single-ring wound protectors, the pooled estimated risk of SSI was 0.31 (95% CI 0.14 to 0.67) times the pooled estimated risk in the control groups. As blinding status of outcome assessors was identified as a significant source of between study heterogeneity, the design of the wound protector as well as the method of outcome classification may be important considerations for the design of future wound protector trials.

According to the actual evidence, it is recommended the use of CWEP devices in clean-contaminated, contaminated and dirty abdominal surgical procedures for the purpose of reducing the rate of SSI.

ADHESIVE DRAPES AND GOWNS

Drapes and gowns are available for single-use or multiple-use, with varying compositions. Adhesive plastic incise drapes are used on a patient's skin after surgical site preparation, with or without antimicrobial impregnation, and the surgeon performs the incision of the drape and the skin simultaneously. In available guidelines, there are confl icting recommendations on the use of plastic adhesive drapes, mainly discouraging their use. There are no recommendations on the use of single-use or reusable drapes and gowns for the purpose of SSI prevention. We did a systematic review to investigate the use of sterile disposable or reusable drapes and surgical gowns, and separately the use of plastic adhesive incises drapes, for the purpose of SSI prevention. Results from non-randomised studies have produced conflicting results about the efficacy of this approach, but no systematic review has been conducted to date to guide clinical practice. A recent meta-analysis [2] of the impact of adhesive drapes on SSI included 5 studies with a total 3082 patients comparing adhesive drapes versus no drape, and 2 with a total 1113 patients comparing iodine-impregnated adhesive drapes versus no drape. SSI rates were higher in the adhesive drape groups; iodine impregnation was not associated with any significant difference in SSI. The WHO also performed a meta-analysis assessing adhesive drapes with and without antiseptic impregnation [14] and found no benefit in terms of SSI between using or not using adhesive drapes. Some allergic reactions occurred with impregnated drapes.

Considering the evidence, including potential issues of availability and costs in low-resource settings and the ecological effect, the expert panel suggested that either sterile disposable non-woven or sterile reusable woven drapes and gowns can be used. However, adhesive incise drapes (with or without antimicrobial properties) should not be used for the purpose of preventing SSI.

ANTIMICROBIAL SKIN SEALANTS

Antimicrobial skin sealants, usually composed of cyanoacrylate, are sterile liquids applied to the skin after skin preparation, ahead of incision; on drying, they form a film that is meant to prevent migration towards the surgical site for several days. The WHO experts performed a meta-analysis of the contribution of antimicrobial skin sealants to prevention of SSI, based on 8 randomized trials and 1 observational study, with a total 1974 patients [14], and found no significant impact compared to standard skin preparation. Cyanoacrylate is a generic term referring to a class of compounds that readily polymerize to create sealants. The first cyanoacrylates were discovered in 1942 when searching for a compound that would form a solid adhesive for weapon development. Noted as a wondrous compound that stuck to everything it came into contact with, it quickly fell out of favor. With time, however, uses for these compounds were reexplored. Perhaps the most well-known, household cyanoacrylate, ethyl-2-cyanoacrylate, is more commonly known as SuperGlue. In 1998, the Food and Drug Administration (FDA) approved another cyanoacrylate, 2-octyl-cyanoacrylate, for use as a surgical incision sealant.

More commonly known by trade names such as Dermabond (Ethicon, Somerville, NJ), this compound readily polymerizes when exposed to skin, blood, or moisture creating a barrier to the migration of bacteria into surgical incisions. Additionally, cytotoxic compounds released by this polymerization reaction exhibit bactericidal properties [18].

A number of studies have tried to ascertain if cyanoacrylates can effectively reduce the rate of SSI. Again, results have been mixed and study subject numbers small making it difficult to make a recommendation supporting the widespread use of this compound for the purpose of reducing SSI, particularly in light of its expense. In 2010, Chambers et al. performed a best evidence review evaluating the use of cyanoacrylate glue on sternal surgical incision infections. In this review, a substantial benefit reducing both superficial and deep surgical incision infections in cardiac surgery was observed when cyanoacrylate was applied post-operatively (4.9% versus 2.1%) or even preoperatively (10.8% versus 2.7% or 7.8% versus 1.1% depending on the study) [19]. Enthusiasm for applying these antimicrobial sealants immediately prior to incision has been particularly observed in the cardiothoracic literature. In 2011, Iyer et al. published a study evaluating patients undergoing cardiac bypass in which saphenous vein harvesting was performed bilaterally. In each patient, one leg was pre-treated with sealant whereas the contralateral leg was not pre-treated. Treated legs developed a 2% incidence of infection, whereas untreated legs became infected in 25% of patients. The study was terminated after 47 patients were enrolled [20]. A larger, randomized trial by von Eckardstein et al. comparing patients who underwent cardiac surgery, allocated 146 patients to pretreatment with cyanoacrylate sealant to sternal and graft harvest sites and 147 patients to no treatment. In this study, there was a 35% relative risk reduction in the rate of SSI in pretreated patients. Furthermore, in subgroup analysis, this study showed an 83% relative risk reduction in obese patients who received pre-treatment [21].

In 2010, Lipp et al. performed a systematic review submitted to the Cochran Database including all randomized trials evaluating the use of cyanoacrylate sealants as a pretreatment of skin incisions. Sufficient evidence supporting the use of such sealants was not found and studies noted to be lacking in rigor and quality [22]. In 2014, Vierhout et al. randomized 47 patients undergoing lower extremity revascularization surgery to closure with cyanoacrylate. Although there was a trend to less SSI (4% vs 9%), this study failed to reach statistical significance [23].

Therefore—also to avoid unnecessary costs—antimicrobial sealants should not be used after surgical site skin preparation for the purpose of reducing SSI.

IMPREGNATED DRESSINGS

The 1999 Guideline for Prevention of Surgical Site Infection is clear in its recommendations for management of post-operative surgical incision dressings stating that surgical incisions should be protected with a sterile occlusive dressing for 24 to 48 h post-operatively [24]. Furthermore, when a dressing must be changed, sterile technique should be employed. Beyond simple sterile dressings, there has been question raised as to the benefit of enhancing dressings with antibacterial agents. In particular, a number of studies have attempted to show improved surgical incision healing and decreased SSI in surgical incisions treated with silver impregnated surgical incision dressings. It has long been believed that silver containing compounds have antibacterial properties. In 2011, the Cochrane Database released a review of sixteen randomized trials employing silver impregnated dressings. Unfortunately, it was noted that these trials were too small and of poor quality. It was concluded that there is no evidence that one type of dressing is better than another. In addition, one study even showed slowed surgical incision healing in patients treated with impregnated dressings. In 2012, Biffi et al. again evaluated the use of silver impregnated dressings in patients undergoing surgery for colorectal cancer. Fifty-eight patients' surgical incisions were covered with silver-impregnated dressings and 54 patients' surgical incisions were covered with standard dry sterile dressings. After a follow-up of 30 days, a trend to fewer surgical site infections were noted in the silver dressing group (15.5% vs 20.4%), but this was not statistically significant [25].

REFERENCES

[1] Hollenbeak CS, Murphy D, Dunagan WC, Fraser VJ. Nonrandom selection and the attributable cost of surgical-site infections. *Infect Control Hosp Epidemiol*. 2002;23(4):177-82.

[2] Webster J, Alghamdi A. Use of plastic adhesive drapes during surgery for preventing surgical site infection. *Cochrane Database Syst Rev.* 2015(4):CD006353.

[3] Williams JA, Oates GD, Brown PP, Burden DW, McCall J, Hutchison AG, et al. Abdominal wound infections and plastic wound guards. *Br J Surg.* 1972;59(2):142-6.

[4] Cheng KP, Roslani AC, Sehha N, Kueh JH, Law CW, Chong HY, et al. ALEXIS O-Ring wound retractor vs conventional wound protection for the prevention of surgical site infections in colorectal resections (1). *Colorectal Dis.* 2012;14(6):e346-51.

[5] Pinkney TD, Calvert M, Bartlett DC, Gheorghe A, Redman V, Dowswell G, et al. Impact of wound edge protection devices on surgical site infection after laparotomy: multicentre randomised controlled trial (ROSSINI Trial). *BMJ.* 2013;347:f4305.

[6] PAYNE JT. An adhesive surgical drape. *Am J Surg.* 1956;91(1):110-2.

[7] Mohan HM, McDermott S, Fenelon L, Fearon NM, O'Connell PR, Oon SF, et al. Plastic wound retractors as bacteriological barriers in gastrointestinal surgery: a prospective multi-institutional trial. *J Hosp Infect.* 2012;81(2):109-13.

[8] Horiuchi T, Tanishima H, Tamagawa K, Sakaguchi S, Shono Y, Tsubakihara H, et al. A wound protector shields incision sites from bacterial invasion. *Surg Infect (*Larchmt). 2010;11(6):501-3.

[9] Horiuchi T, Tanishima H, Tamagawa K, Matsuura I, Nakai H, Shouno Y, et al. Randomized, controlled investigation of the anti-infective properties of the Alexis retractor/protector of incision sites. *J Trauma.* 2007;62(1):212-5.

[10] Reid K, Pockney P, Draganic B, Smith SR. Barrier wound protection decreases surgical site infection in open elective colorectal surgery: a randomized clinical trial. *Dis Colon Rectum.* 2010;53(10):1374-80.

[11] Mihaljevic AL, Müller TC, Kehl V, Friess H, Kleeff J. Wound edge protectors in open abdominal surgery to reduce surgical site infections: a systematic review and meta-analysis. *PLoS One.* 2015;10(3):e0121187.

[12] Leaper D, Burman-Roy S, Palanca A, Cullen K, Worster D, Gautam-Aitken E, et al. Prevention and treatment of surgical site infection: summary of NICE guidance. *BMJ*. 2008;337:a1924.

[13] Anderson DJ, Podgorny K, Berríos-Torres SI, Bratzler DW, Dellinger EP, Greene L, et al. Strategies to prevent surgical site infections in acute care hospitals: 2014 update. *Infect Control Hosp Epidemiol*. 2014;35 Suppl 2:S66-88.

[14] Leaper DJ, Edmiston CE. World Health Organization: global guidelines for the prevention of surgical site infection. *J Hosp Infect*. 2017;95(2):135-6.

[15] Psaila JV, Wheeler MH, Crosby DL. The role of plastic wound drapes in the prevention of wound infection following abdominal surgery. *Br J Surg*. 1977;64(10):729-32.

[16] Gheorghe A, Calvert M, Pinkney TD, Fletcher BR, Bartlett DC, Hawkins WJ, et al. Systematic review of the clinical effectiveness of wound-edge protection devices in reducing surgical site infection in patients undergoing open abdominal surgery. *Ann Surg*. 2012;255(6):1017-29.

[17] Edwards JP, Ho AL, Tee MC, Dixon E, Ball CG. Wound protectors reduce surgical site infection: a meta-analysis of randomized controlled trials. *Ann Surg*. 2012;256(1):53-9.

[18] de Almeida Manzano RP, Naufal SC, Hida RY, Guarnieri LO, Nishiwaki-Dantas MC. Antibacterial analysis in vitro of ethyl-cyanoacrylate against ocular pathogens. *Cornea*. 2006;25(3):350-1.

[19] Chambers A, Scarci M. Is skin closure with cyanoacrylate glue effective for the prevention of sternal wound infections? *Interact Cardiovasc Thorac Surg*. 2010;10(5):793-6.

[20] Iyer A, Gilfillan I, Thakur S, Sharma S. Reduction of surgical site infection using a microbial sealant: a randomized trial. *J Thorac Cardiovasc Surg*. 2011;142(2):438-42.

[21] von Eckardstein AS, Lim CH, Dohmen PM, Pêgo-Fernandes PM, Cooper WA, Oslund SG, et al. A randomized trial of a skin sealant to reduce the risk of incision contamination in cardiac surgery. *Ann Thorac Surg*. 2011;92(2):632-7.

[22] Lipp A, Phillips C, Harris P, Dowie I. Cyanoacrylate microbial sealants for skin preparation prior to surgery. *Cochrane Database Syst Rev.* 2013(8):CD008062.

[23] Vierhout BP, Ott A, Reijnen MM, Oskam J, van den Dungen JJ, Zeebregts CJ. Cyanoacrylate skin microsealant for preventing surgical site infection after vascular surgery: a discontinued randomized clinical trial. *Surg Infect* (Larchmt). 2014;15(4):425-30.

[24] Mangram AJ, Horan TC, Pearson ML, Silver LC, Jarvis WR. Guideline for Prevention of Surgical Site Infection, 1999. Centers for Disease Control and Prevention (CDC) Hospital Infection Control Practices Advisory Committee. *Am J Infect Control.* 1999;27(2):97-132; quiz 3-4; discussion 96.

[25] Biffi R, Fattori L, Bertani E, Radice D, Rotmensz N, Misitano P, et al. Surgical site infections following colorectal cancer surgery: a randomized prospective trial comparing common and advanced antimicrobial dressing containing ionic silver. *World J Surg Oncol.* 2012;10:94.

In: Prophylaxis of Surgical Site Infection …   ISBN: 978-1-53615-615-7
Editors: Jaime Ruiz-Tovar et al.   © 2019 Nova Science Publishers, Inc.

Chapter 9

WOUND IRRIGATION

Gilberto González Ramírez[*] *MD*

Universidad de Guadalajara Jalisco, México
Department of Surgery and Bariatric Surgery,
Centro Medico Puerta de Hierro, Guadalajara Jalisco, México

ABSTRACT

There are different challenges in the course of a surgery treatment. These go from the type of surgical procedure until the adequate close of the incision. In this scenario, the wound needs an environment that gives the best or almost the best conditions for normal healing. In such conditions, to avoid surgical site infection (SSI) at the time of the surgery or later and to keep clean the wound is one of the main factors to achieve a good environment with the sequence of hormonal activation and inflammatory response, stimulating the regeneration of the tissue with a properly closure. In this chapter, we will talk about the wound irrigation, the different type of solutions to do it, which one is more effective and why in our opinion, and which is the actual consensus about this practice. There are several opinions and different experiences around the world, sometimes more supported by evidence and other not so much.

---

[*] Corresponding Author's Email: gilpchmd@yahoo.com.mx.

Keywords: wound irrigation, wound management, surgical site infection, incision, solutions, healing, clousure

INTRODUCTION

Despite extensive scrutiny, multiple collaborative efforts, and significant advances in infection prevention practices, approximately 500,000 surgical site infections (SSIs), with an associated cost estimated at $10 billion, occur annually in the United States alone [1, 2].

At the 2013 annual Association for Professionals in Infection Control and Epidemiology conference, a focus group of key thought leaders in infection prevention and epidemiology, including epidemiologists, surgeons, and infection prevention directors for major health care systems, convened to address the implications of different surgical irrigation practices. The group agreed that, in an era where health care-associated infections rank as the fifth leading cause of death [3] and carry an attributable per patient cost ranging from $80,000 to $110,000 [4, 5], closer investigation of surgical irrigation practices, as an integral part of the infection prevention process, is warranted [1].

A complete wound history along with anatomic and specific medical considerations for each patient provides the basis of decision making for wound management. It is essential to apply an evidence-based approach and consider each wound individually in order to create the optimal conditions for wound healing [6].

Without proper cleansing and wound care, these acute wounds can lead to complications, such as poor healing and infection. Optimizing wound healing through proper acute wound management involves removal of harmful debris/necrotic tissue, exploration for underlying injuries, control of bacterial burden and appropriate closure [6].

BACKGROUND

Surgical Site Infection

Postoperative surgical site infection (SSI) represents as one of the most frequent complications following abdominal surgery. In the USA, an estimated 300,000 to 500,000 cases of SSI occur annually [8, 24]. Similar figures are reported from Germany [7, 9], the UK [10], and France [11]. The incidence of SSI varies substantially, depending on the type and site of surgery [8]. According to recent high-level randomized controlled trials (RCTs) with standardized SSI definitions, rates range from around 15% (BaFo trial [12]; PROUD trial [13] up to 25% (ROSSINI trial) [14] following laparotomy for visceral surgery. SSIs contribute substantially to postoperative morbidity and mortality and have been shown to significantly increase the mean length of hospital stay and treatment costs [11, 15, 24]. Therefore, measures to prevent SSI are urgently needed [16].

Surgical site infections are recognized as a common surgical complication, occurring in about 3% of all surgical procedures and in up to 20% of patients undergoing emergency intra-abdominal procedures [17, 18].

Surgical site infections (SSIs) are an adverse outcome of surgery accounting for the majority of healthcare- associated infections around the world [20, 21]. In developing countries, more than one in ten of all surgical procedures is complicated by an SSI [22]. Although the overall risk of SSIs is much lower in developed countries, they remain a serious threat to patient safet [20, 21]. Such infections increase morbidity and mortality rates and prolong hospital stays [19, 20, 23, 24].

Many factors have been associated with the risk of SSI, and consequently, a range of preventive measures has been proposed. One of these is prophylactic intra-operative wound irrigation (pIOWI), a seemingly simple intervention defined by the flow of a solution across the surface of an open wound to achieve tissue hydration. It removes and dilutes body fluids, bacteria, and cellular debris and additionally may have a bactericidal effect when additives, such as antibiotics or antiseptic agents are used (see Table 1 for an overview of the definitions used). As many as 97% of surgeons commonly practice IOWI [25, 26]. Nonetheless, it is not part of general practice in every country or hospital. Moreover, methods differ depending on the patient population, surface of application, technique, and solutions used. Similar variations in methods and results can be observed in studies investigating the effect of IOWI [18, 27, 28].

Table 1. Systematic review and meta-analysis of randomized controlled trials evaluating prophylactic intra-operative wound irrigation for the prevention of surgical site infections Stijn W. de Jonge,[1,*] Surgical Infections Volume 18, Number 4, 2017 a Mary Ann Liebert, Inc. DOI: 10.1089/sur.2016.272 [19]

Prophylactic intra-operative wound irrigation (pIOWI)	The flow of a solution across the surface of an open wound to achieve wound hydration. It physically removes and dilutes body fluids, bacteria, and cellular debris and has a bactericidal effect when additives such as antibiotics or antiseptic agents are used
Intra-operative wound irrigation as therapeutic intervention	CDC wound class IV was considered a pre-existent infection; irrigation field was considered to be therapeutic, not prophylactic
Intra-operative wound irrigation as prophylactic intervention	CDC wound class I–III was considered potentially contaminated; irrigation was considered to be prophylactic Irrigation of the newly made incision was always considered prophylactic, regardless of the wound classification, as the incision did not exist prior to the procedure and established infection was impossible.
Syringe pressure irrigation	Solution delivered with a syringe with an intravenous catheter applying force by hand.
Pulse pressure irrigation	Irrigation with a mechanical device that delivers pulsatile saline irrigation.
US Centers for Disease Control and Prevention (CDC) surgical wound classification	**Class I/Clean:** An uninfected operative wound in which no inflammation is encountered and the respiratory, alimentary, genital, or uninfected urinary tract is not entered. In addition, clean sites are closed primarily and, if necessary, drained with closed drainage. Operative incisions that follow non-penetrating (blunt) trauma should be included in this category if they meet the criteria. **Class II/Clean–Contaminated:** An operative wound in which the respiratory, alimentary, genital, or urinary tracts are entered under controlled conditions and without unusual contamination. Specifically, operations involving the biliary tract, appendix, vagina, and oropharynx are included in this category, provided no evidence of infection or major break in technique is encountered. **Class III/Contaminated:** Open, fresh, accidental wounds. In addition, operations with major breaks in sterile technique (e.g., open cardiac massage) or gross spillage from the gastrointestinal tract, and incisions in which acute, nonpurulent inflammation is encountered, are included in this category. **Class IV/Dirty–Infected:** Old traumatic wounds with retained devitalized tissue and those that involve existing clinical infection or perforated viscera. This definition suggests that the organisms causing postoperative infection were present in the operative field before the operation.

Among the available guidelines on SSI prevention, few have addressed the topic of IOWI and give contradictory recommendations. The guidelines from the United Kingdom National Institute for Health and Care Excellence (NICE), issued in 2008 and updated in 2013, advised against IOWI and intra-peritoneal lavage [29]. In contrast, the 2014 guidelines of the Society for Healthcare Epidemiology of America (SHEA) and the Infectious Diseases Society of America (IDSA) recommend using antiseptic incision lavage [28]. Many of the solutions commonly used for irrigation are not licensed for open incisions by the U.S. Food and Drug Administration [18, 28, 30].

Infection may occur within the surgical site at any depth, starting from the skin itself and extending to the deepest cavity that remains after resection of an organ. Superficial SSI involves tissues down to the fascia (Figure 1), whereas deep SSI extends beneath the fascia but not intracavitary. Organ/space infections are subfascial or intracavitary, but if related directly to an operation, are considered to be SSIs [18].

Cellulitis is infection-related erythema of skin (although other tissues may be affected) without drainage or fluctuance. Abscess refers to localized collections of purulent material within tissue. Necrotizing soft tissue infections (NSTIs) invade tissue widely and rapidly, causing widespread tissue necrosis. When fascia is involved, the infection is referred to correctly as necrotizing fasciitis [18].

Bacteria's Biofilm

The importance of biofilm formation as an element of wound infection has recently been stressed [31]. When bacteria proliferate in wounds, they form microcolonies, which attach to the wound bed and secrete a glycocalyx, or any kind of extracellular matrix, and take up an interdependent surface-attached existence. These microbial communities, called 'biofilms,' protect the organisms against antibiotics, antiseptics and host immune defences [32]. Almost all bacterial species form biofilm in vivo [33], thus representing a therapeutic challenge in many, if not most, bacterial diseases. Biofilm formation has also been linked to the emergence of a variety of opportunistic pathogens, such as *Staphylococcus epidermidis* and *Pseudomonas aeruginosa,* which contribute to persistent infections by changing environmental parameters [34, 84].

Definitions

Primary closure, also known as healing by first intention, represents closure of a wound at the time of initial presentation. Wound edges are approximated with suture, adhesives, staples, or strips after appropriate wound management techniques are applied.

Delayed primary closure represents a delay in wound closure for approximately 3–5 days. This is ideal for delayed presentations or for wound infection concerns. If there are no signs of infection and the wound margins appear healthy, removal of devitalized tissue and subsequent primary closure is appropriate.

Healing by secondary intention represents those wounds that are allowed to heal through contraction—a natural, unaided physiologic property. While appropriate wound management practices are involved, no attempt is made to aid wound closure [6].

Clean surgical procedures are those where the operation has affected only integumentary and musculoskeletal soft tissues. Clean- contaminated procedures are those where a hollow viscus (eg, alimentary, biliary, genitourinary, respiratory tract) has been opened under controlled circumstances (eg, elective colon surgery). Contaminated procedures are those where bacteria has been introduced extensively into a normally sterile body cavity, but for a period of time too brief to allow infection to become established during surgery (eg, penetrating abdominal trauma, enterotomy during adhesiolysis for mechanical bowel obstruction). Dirty procedures are those where the surgery is performed to control established infection (eg, colon resection for complicated diverticulitis) [18].

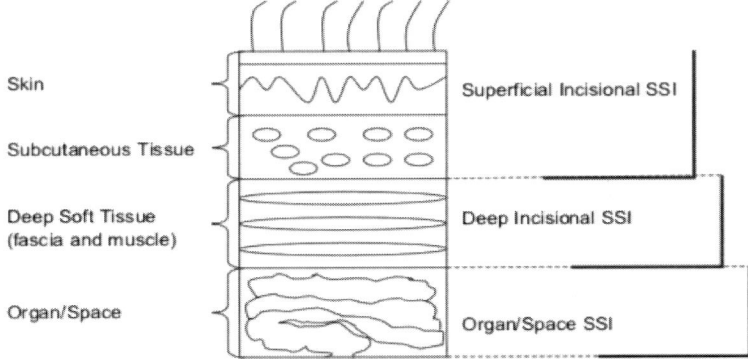

Figure 1. Surgical site infections. (Adapted from Mangram AJ, Horan TC, Pearson ML, et al. The Hospital Infection Control Practices Advisory Committee. Guideline for the prevention of surgical site infection, 1999. Infect Control Hosp Epidemiol 1999; 20:247-80).

Normal acute wounds usually progress through an orderly sequential trajectory of hemostasis, proliferation, maturation, and remodeling [35]. After initial injury to the dermal tissue, hemostasis is established by platelet aggregation, fibrin clot formation, and the subsequent coagulation pathways. Local migration of neutrophils and macrophages initiates an acute inflammatory response to help prevent microbial overgrowth as well as initiate wound healing. During the proliferative phase, deficiencies in soft tissue are replaced with healthy new granulation tissue and matrix material. As healing progresses, the majority of type III collagen formed by fibroblasts is converted to type I collagen to enhance soft tissue strength and integrity [6, 36].

To ensure the normal physiology of healing, wounds must have sufficient blood supply. Inflammation, infection, or residual debris may delay or prevent adequate healing. As healing occurs, wound tensile strength will approach 20% at 3 weeks and 60% by 4 months [6, 35].

The primary goals for wound care are to attain a functional closure, decrease potential risk for infection, and minimize scar formation [6, 37].

Proper wound preparation improves healing and outcomes. While evidence-based recommendations for wound care exist, many practitioners continue to treat wounds based on personal preference—some employing unnecessary or possibly detrimental techniques [6, 38].

Pressure Irrigation

Wound irrigation is arguably the most important step for optimizing wound healing as long as there is sufficient pressure and volume. Irrigation pressure recommendations that are often cited in the literature come mostly from studies in chronic wounds (such as pressure ulcers). Many studies either failed to describe how pressure was measured or identify the actual realized pressure on the tissues. Within the realm of acute wound management, the term 'high pressure' irrigation is frequently used to describe the best practice for wound irrigation. However, it is important to understand that this term reflects a wide range of pressures and a paucity of well-supported literature as to the deliverable irrigant pressure [6].

Classically, equipment used for irrigation has included bulb syringes, syringes with an attached needle or catheter, intravenous or irrigation fluid in plastic containers with a pour cap or nozzle, and pressure canisters. Puncturing containers of irrigation fluid and manually squeezing are inadequate for pressure irrigation [39]. Studies have shown that when using a syringe with an attached 19-gauge needle, pressures range from 11 to 31 psi—however, only 8 psi may reach the wound [39, 40]. Current medical devices have been designed to provide a more consistent and measurable application of wound irrigation pressure. Clinicians currently believe that these advances may provide a better approach to wound cleansing [6, 41].

There is some evidence that very high pressure irrigation may actually increase infection rates due to further tissue damage. This is particularly evident in highly vascularized wounds, such as the face and scalp [6, 42].

A study by Chisholm found no difference in infection rates of lacerations that required closures when irrigation was done using a pressure canister compared to a syringe/needle irrigation (5.0% vs. 3.6%; $P = 0.05$) [43]. Longmire found that high pressures of 13 psi, generated by using a needle and syringe, were effective in reducing inflammation and infection when compared to irrigation using a bulb syringe associated with lower pressures [40]. Pressures of 8–12 psi in the wound are believed to overcome the adhesive forces of the introduced bacterium [40, 43].

However, both of these studies were limited by the inability to measure consistent pressures across the tissue beds being irrigated [6].

Irrigation Volume

Irrigation volumes of 50 to 100 ml per cm of laceration length have been reported [44, 43]. The volume of irrigation should be adjusted to the wound characteristics and degree of contamination. All wound surfaces should be irrigated and may require pulling open the wound edges and flaps for exposure [44]. Repeat irrigation has been recommended after any re-examination of the wound [6, 45].

Irrigation Solution

Decontamination, including brushing off any dry chemicals prior to copious irrigation, is an essential part of the initial wound management. It is important to consider toxicological exposure as it relates to wound irrigation. Antiseptic solutions, such as povidone-iodine, chlorhexidine, and hydrogen peroxide, are toxic to tissues and may impede acute wound healing [41]. The current literature supports no difference in ED wound infection rates when using potable tap water versus saline in adult and pediatric populations [46]. Further, studies comparing saline irrigation with diluted 1% povidone-iodine have shown no difference in infection rates [43, 47, 48]. A study of chemical burns (N = 24) recommended copious amounts of potable tap water or saline for irrigation and decontamination [6, 49].

There are 3 critical variables in the surgical irrigation process: delivery, volume, and solution additives. In the absence of formal guidelines, anecdotal evidence suggests that a wide variety of practices are used with regard to each of these three variables [1].

Delivery

Surgical irrigation delivery includes choosing delivery method, pressure (the American College of Surgeons [ACS] defines high pressure as 15 to 35 psi and low pressure as 1 to 15 psi [50], and continuous or pulsatile flow. Neither the ACS nor the Association of periOperative Registered Nurses (AORN) has published practice recommendations on surgical irrigation delivery [1].

A number of studies have been performed to evaluate optimal pressures for wound irrigation. The majority of these have shown high-pressure irrigation to be most effective in bacteria and foreign material removal; however, high-pressure irrigation has also been associated with impairment of the local immune response, tissue damage, and propagation of bacteria deeper into tissue or bone [51]. These negative effects suggest that high-pressure lavage should be limited to conditions where contamination is severe and the anticipated difficulty in bacterial removal outweighs the potential of propagation of bacteria [51]. Whereas no official guidelines exist for optimal pressures, recommendations have suggested utilizing pressures of 8 to 12 psi in traumatic wounds in an effort to overcome the adhesive forces of bacteria [1, 52].

Volume

Similar to the lack of data on delivery of surgical irrigation, there are no official recommendations on irrigant fluid volumes [51]. Additionally, there are no published human studies. Animal studies have indicated that increasing volume improves bacteria and foreign material removal to a point, but excessive volume also reduces the concentration of beneficial cytokines involved in the correct healing procedure. Thus, optimal volumes remain undefined [1, 51, 53].

Additives

Over the years, however, a variety of different additives, commonly grouped into the categories of antibiotics, surfactants, and antiseptics, have been combined with irrigation fluids in an attempt to optimize infection prevention. Unfortunately, there are few well-designed clinical trials looking at these practices and, hence, no established clinical guideline [1, 54].

Intraoperative Wound Irrigation (IOWI)

Intraoperative wound irrigation is the flow of a solution across the surface of an open wound to achieve wound hydration and it is widely practised to help prevent SSI [55, 56]. It is intended to act as a physical cleaner by removing cellular debris, surface bacteria and body fluids, to have a diluting effect on possible contamination, and to function as a local antibacterial agent when an antiseptic or antibiotic agent is used. Up to 97% of surgeons state that they use intraoperative irrigation [55, 57].

However, practices vary depending on the patient population, the surface of application and solutions used. Similar variations in methodology and results can be observed in studies investigating the effect of wound irrigation [57, 58].

Results Forty-one RCTs reporting primary data of over 9000 patients were analyzed. Meta-analysis on the effect of IOWI with any solution compared to no irrigation revealed a significant benefit in the reduction of SSI rates (OR = 0.54, 95% confidence Interval (CI) [0.42; 0.69], $p < 0.0001$) [16].

Meta-analysis showed a significant benefit of IOWI with any solution in comparison to no irrigation [16].

Further, sub-group analysis showed that the estimated effect in reduction of postoperative SSI was significant only for IOWI with topical antibiotics or PVP-I but not for saline [16].

IOWI with Saline

Plain saline is a widely used irrigation solution, as it is isotonic and does not interfere with wound healing [59]. Furthermore, it is generally used to clean wounds from blood clots and necrotic tissue. However, evidence for IOWI with saline to prevent SSI is scarce. Only three RCTs comparing saline with no irrigation were identified [60, 61, 62], and meta-analysis showed no statistically significant effect on the rate of SSIs (Figure 4c, OR = 0.64, 95% CI [0.28; 1.46], p = 0.29) [16].

IOWI with PVP-I

Much debate has also surfaced over the use of PVP-I, and the use of this solution has been removed from many wound management regimes because of a putative negative effect on tissue regeneration. PVP-I demonstrates dose-dependent levels of tissue toxicity but is still better tolerated than preparations containing chlorhexidine or octenidine [63]. However, when studied in a clinical context, a recent evidence-based review of the effects of PVP-I solutions on wound healing failed to show a negative effect [64]. Consequently, the ma- jority of high-quality trials analyzed in that review supported the use of PVP-I for IOWI. The NICE guidelines do not recommend the use of IOWI or intra-operative skin redisinfection with PVP-I products [10, 16, 65]. Nevertheless, the recently published recommendations for SSI prophylaxis by the World Health Organization (WHO) recommend its use at at a 10% concentration, diluted in plain saline [83].

IOWI with Topical Antibiotics

In clinical practice, IOWI with solutions containing antibiotics used to be widespread in the 1980s, especially in dirty-contaminated abdominal or trauma/orthopedic surgery [66]. Currently, guidelines do not support the use of antibiotic IOWI anymore, due to the lack of evidence for their benefit and the potential enhancement of microbial resistance [10, 16].

Especially in obese patients, who are predisposed to develop SSI, infusion of topical antibiotics to the wound allowed to achieve higher local concentrations in the poorly perfused subcutaneous adipose tissue than by intravenous application [67]. In line with this data, a significant reduction of SSIs in this subgroup analysis of 19 trials comparing IOWI with antibiotic solutions vs. no irrigation (Figure 4a; OR = 0.39, 95% CI [0.27; 0.55], p < 0.0001). However, different antibiotics, concentrations, and applications were used meaning that heterogeneity was high and no regime can currently be recommended unequivocally [16].

HOWEVER IN ONE META-ANALYSIS THE AUTHORS CONSIDERED...

Evidence of low quality shows that prophylactic incisional irrigation with aqueous PVP-I solution has a significant benefit on the SSI rate, particularly in clean and clean- contaminated wounds. No dose–response effect was detected. Referring to incisional irrigation with saline, evidence of moderate to very low quality shows a significant effect on SSI rate when applied with force or using pulse pressure, but not with regular irrigation. There is no significant benefit to the use of antibiotic solutions for prophylactic incisional wound irrigation or for the use of pIOWI in the abdomen or mediastinum [19].

The most commonly used irrigation solution is saline followed by aqueous PVP-I or anti- biotic solutions [68, 69, 70]. The efficacy and clinical safety of irrigation with these solutions has been the subject of debate [19, 71, 72].

Wound irrigation using aqueous chlorhexidine (CHX) may be an alternative when extrapolating the favourable results from alcohol-based CHX used for pre-operative skin preparation, but clinical data are lacking. The results of aqueous 0.05% chlorhexidine gluconate as a wound irrigation fluid in the laboratory and animal studies are promising [19, 73, 74].

Charles E. Edmiston Et al. they considered the CHG (clorhexidine glouconato), as other alternative to wound irrigation, and they consider ... A new focus for the use of CHG in surgical patients involves irrigation of the wound prior to closure with 0.05% CHG followed by saline rinse. Recent laboratory studies suggest that, following a 1-minute exposure, 0.05% CHG produces a >5-log reduction against selective health care-associated pathogens and reduces microbial adherence to the surface of implantable biomedical devices [75].

STATEMENTS OF DIFFERENT SCIENTIFIC SOCIETIES ABOUT WOUND IRRIGATION

World Health Organization

- The panel considers that there is insufficient evidence to recommend for or against saline irrigation of incisional wounds before closure for the purpose of preventing SSI [57]
- The panel suggests considering the use of irrigation of the incisional wound with an aqueous PVP-I solution before closure for the purpose of preventing SSI, particularly in clean and clean-contaminated wounds [57]
- The panel suggests that antibiotic incisional wound irrigation before closure should not be used for the purpose of preventing SSI. *(Conditional recommendations/low quality of evidence)* [57]

Centers for Disease Control and Prevention. Guideline for the Prevention of Surgical Site Infection, 2017

- 9A. Consider intraoperative irrigation of deep or subcutaneous tissues with aqueous iodophor solution for the prevention of SSI. Intraperitoneal lavage with aqueous iodophor solution in contaminated or dirty abdominal procedures is not necessary. (Category II–weak recommendation; moderate-quality evidence suggesting a trade-off between clinical benefits and harms.) [76]
- 10. Randomized controlled trial evidence was insufficient to evaluate the trade offs between the benefits and harms of repeat application of antiseptic agents to the patient's skin immediately before closing the surgical incision for the prevention of SSI. (No recom- mendation/unresolved issue) [76].

World Health Organization. Global Guidelines for the Prevention of Surgical Site Infection

Saline wound irrigation: There is insufficient evidence to recommend for or against saline irrigation of incisional wounds for the purpose of preventing SSI [77].

Povidone iodine irrigation: Consider the use of irrigation of the incisional wound with an aqueous povidone iodine solution before closure for the purpose of preventing SSI, particularly in clean and clean-contaminated wounds [77].

Antibiotic irrigation: Antibiotic incisional wound irrigation before closure should not be used for the purpose of preventing SSI [77].

There are a homogeneous consensus, however still a lack of randomized trials in the actual literature.

GENERAL CONCLUSION

High-quality evidence from future RCTs using standardized outcome parameters is awaited urgently to clearly establish the role of IOWI in abdominal surgery on an evidence-based level in order to encounter the substantial problem of this huge health care burden worldwide [16].

Wound irrigation remains controversial as a means of reducing the risk of SSI. There is little information to suggest that routine low-pressure washing of an incision with saline reduces the risk of SSI [78], but high pressure (ie, pulse-irrigation) may be beneficial [79]. An increasing body of knowledge suggests that topical antibiotics placed into the incision during surgery can minimize the risk of SSI [80, 81], but it might be desirable to accomplish the same result with topical antiseptics rather than antibiotics to minimize the possibility of the development of resistance [18].

Josie Chundamala et al. In their conclusions they said:

> In conclusion, the evidence suggests that povidone-iodine irrigation may be effective in preventing surgical site infection. However, more studies, especially double-blind RCTs, should be conducted to determine the "ideal" solution of povidone-iodine irrigation as well as specific risks associated with its use [82].

CONCLUSION

In our experience, we consider that the irrigation of the wound with saline solution plays a role for intraoperative cleaning the wound of detritus, residual material, fibrine, clots or even intraluminal gastric or intestinal content. However, there is insufficient evidence to support its isolated use for prevention of SSI. The wound irrigation with a pvp-i solution has demonstrated more evidence as preventive measure, mainly in clean or clean-contaminated procedures. In more contaminated areas, there is not enough evidence to establish a strong recommendation, but it makes sense to apply this measure also in contaminated or dirty surgeries, as it may only represent a benefit. There is no evidence of adverse effects or development of bacterial resistance associated with its use.

On the other hand, we do not recomended the addition of antibiotic in the solution for irrigation. Actual evidence has demonstrated that antibiotics do not imply a further reduction in SSI rate than that of pvp-i solutions, and represent a risk for development of bacterial resistances. There is some evidence that topical antibiotic may be beneficial in obese patients, but further studies must be conducted to clarify this item.

In conclusion, volume, pressure and addition of drugs are items that still remain controversial. More randomized trials in these issues are necessary to get more evidence-based experience.

REFERENCES

[1] Surgical wound irrigation: A call for evidence-based standardization of practice Sue Barnes RN, BSN, CIC, Maureen Spencer RN, MEd, CIC, Denise Graham, Helen Boehm Johnson MD, *American Journal of Infection Control* 42 (2014) 525-9.

[2] Anderson DJ, Kaye KS, Classen D, Arias KM, Podgorny K, Burstin H, et al. Strategies to prevent surgical site infections in acute care hospitals. *Infect Control Hosp Epidemiol* 2008;29:551-61.

[3] Stone PW. Economic burden of healthcare-associated infections: an American perspective. Expert Rev Pharmacoeconomics *Outcomes Res* 2009;9:417-22.

[4] Tubaki VR, Rajasekaran S, Shetty AP. Effects of using intravenous antibiotic only versus local intrawound vancomycin antibiotic powder application in addition to intravenous antibiotics on postoperative infection in spine surgery in 907 patients. *Spine* 2013;38:2149-55.

[5] Greco G, Shi W, Michler R, Blackstone E, Kron I, Moquete E, et al. *The economic impact of healthcare associated infections in cardiac surgery*. 2013. Accessed December 30, 2013.

[6] Acute wound management: revisiting the approach to assessment, irrigation, and closure considerations Bret A. Nicks & Elizabeth A. Ayello & Kevin Woo & Diane Nitzki-George & R. Gary Sibbald Received: 26 April 2010 / Accepted: 30 June 2010 / Published online: 27 August 2010 # Springer-Verlag London Ltd 2010 *Int J Emerg Med* (2010) 3:399–407 DOI 10.1007/s12245-010-0217-5.

[7] Gastmeier P, Brandt C, Sohr D, Babikir R, Mlageni D, Daschner F et al. (2004) Postoperative Wundinfektionen nach stationären und ambulanten Operationen [Postoperative wound infections after inpatient and outpatient operations]. *Bundesgesundheitsbl Gesundheitsforsch Gesundheitsschutz* 47(4):339–344. doi:10.1007/s00103-004-0805-8.

[8] de Lissovoy G, Fraeman K, Hutchins V, Murphy D, Song D, Vaughn BB (2009) Surgical site infection: incidence and impact on hospital utilization and treatment costs. *Am J Infect Control* 37(5):387–397. doi:10.1016/j.ajic.2008.12.010.

[9] Geffers C (2011) *Postoperative Wundinfektionen* [*Postoperative wound infections*]. Institut für Hygiene und Umweltmedizin der Charité, Berlin.

[10] National Institute for Health and Clinical Excellence (NICE) (2008) Surgical site infection—prevention and treatment of surgical site infection. *NICE Clinical Guideline* 74. RCGO, London.

[11] Lamarsalle L, Hunt B, Schauf M, Szwarcensztein K, Valentine WJ (2013) Evaluating the clinical and economic burden of healthcare-associated infections during hospitalization for surgery in France. *Epidemiol Infect* 141(12):2473–2482. doi:10.1017/ s09502688130 00253.

[12] Mihaljevic AL, Schirren R, Ozer M, Ottl S, Grun S, Michalski CW et al. (2014) Multicenter double-blinded randomized controlled trial of standard abdominal wound edge protection with surgical dressings versus coverage with a sterile circular polyethylene drape for prevention of surgical site infections: a CHIR-Net Trial (BaFO; NCT01181206). *Ann Surg* 260(5):730–739. doi:10.1097/SLA. 000 0000000000954.

[13] Diener MK, Knebel P, Kieser M, Schuler P, Schiergens TS, Atanassov V et al. (2014) Effectiveness of triclosan-coated PDS Plus versus uncoated PDS II sutures for prevention of surgical site infection after abdominal wall closure: the randomised controlled PROUD trial. *Lancet* 384(9938):142–152. doi:10.1016/S0140- 6736 (14)60238-5.

[14] Pinkney TD, Calvert M, Bartlett DC, Gheorghe A, Redman V, Dowswell G et al. (2013) Impact of wound edge protection devices on surgical site infection after laparotomy: multicentre randomised controlled trial (ROSSINI Trial). *BMJ* 347:f4305. doi:10.1136/bmj. f4305.

[15] Merle V, Germain JM, Chamouni P, Daubert H, Froment L, Michot F et al. (2000) Assessment of prolonged hospital stay attributable to surgical site infections using appropriateness evaluation protocol. *Am J Infect Control* 28(2):109–115.

[16] Intra-operative wound irrigation to reduce surgical site infections after abdominal surgery: a systematic review and meta-analysis Tara C. Mueller & Martin Loos & Bernhard Haller & André L. Mihaljevic & Ulrich Nitsche & Dirk Wilhelm & Helmut Friess & Jörg Kleeff & Franz G. Bader Received: 22 September 2014 / Accepted: 1 February 2015 / Published online: 14 February 2015 # Springer-Verlag Berlin Heidelberg 2015 Langenbecks *Arch Surg* (2015) 400:167–181 DOI 10.1007/s00423-015-1279-x.

[17] Barie PS. Surgical site infections: Epidemiology and prevention. *Surg Infect* (Larchmt)2002; 3(Suppl 1):S9–21.

[18] Surgical Site Infections Philip S. Barie, MD, MBA[*], Soumitra R. Eachempati, MD. Division of Critical Care and Trauma, Department of Surgery P713A, Weill Medical College of Cornell University, 525 East 68 Street, New York, NY 10021, USA. *Surg Clin N Am* 85 (2005) 1115–1135.

[19] Systematic Review and Meta-Analysis of Randomized Controlled Trials Evaluating Prophylactic Intra-Operative Wound Irrigation for the Prevention of Surgical Site Infections Stijn W. de Jonge,[1,*]

Surgical Infections Volume 18, Number 4, 2017 a Mary Ann Liebert, Inc. DOI: 10.1089/sur.2016.272.

[20] Magill SS, Edwards JR, Bamberg W, et al. Multistate point-prevalence survey of health care-associated infec- tions. *N Engl J Med* 2014;370:1198–1208.

[21] Gris˘kevic˘iene J. European Centre for Disease Prevention and Control. *Surveillance of Surgical Site Infections in Europe 2010–2011.* Stockholm. ECDC. 2013.

[22] Allegranzi B, Bagheri Nejad S, Combescure C, et al. Burden of endemic health-care-associated infection in de- veloping countries: Systematic review and meta-analysis. *Lancet* 2011;377:228–241.

[23] De Lissovoy G, Fraeman K, Hutchins V, et al. Surgical site infection: Incidence and impact on hospital utilization and treatment costs. *Am J Infect Control* 2009;37:387–397.

[24] Kirkland KB, Briggs JP, Trivette SL, Wilkinson WE, Sexton DJ (1999) The impact of surgical-site infections in the 1990s: attribut- able mortality, excess length of hospitalization, and extra costs. *Infect Control Hosp Epidemiol* 20(11):725–730. doi:10.1086/501572.

[25] Whiteside OJ, Tytherleigh MG, Thrush S, et al. Intra- operative peritoneal lavage: Who does it and why? *Ann R Coll Surg Engl* 2005;87:255–258.

[26] Pivot D, Tiv M, Luu M, et al. Survey of intraoperative povidone–iodine application to prevent surgical site infec- tion in a French region. *J Hosp Infect* 2011;77:363–364.

[27] Raymond DP, Pelletier SJ, Crabtree TD, et al. Surgicalinfection and the age in population. *Am Surg* 2001;67:827–32.

[28] Pomposelli JJ, Baxter JK III, Babineau TJ, et al. Early postoperative glucose control predicts nosocomial infection rate in diabetic patients. *JPEN J Parenter Enteral Nutr* 1998;22:77–81.

[29] Latham R, Lancaster AD, Covington JF, et al. The association of diabetes and glucose control with surgical-site infections among cardiothoracic surgery patients. *Infect Control Hosp Epidemiol* 2001;22:607–12.

[30] Delgado-Rodriguez M, Medina-Cuadros M, Martinez-Gallego G, et al. Total cholesterol, HDL cholesterol, and risk of nosocomial infection: a prospective study in surgical patients. *Infect Control Hosp Epidemiol* 1997;18:9–18.

[31] James GA, Swogger E, Wolcott R, Pulcini ED, Secor P, Sestrich J, Costerton JW, Stew- art PS: Biofilms in chronic wounds. *Wound Repair Regen* 2008;16:37–44.

[32] Lewis K: Riddle of biofilm resistance. *Anti- microb Agents Chemother* 2001;45:999– 1007.

[33] Jefferson KK: What drives bacteria to pro- duce a biofilm? *FEMS Microbiol Lett* 2004; 236:163–173.

[34] Evaluation of the Efficacy and Tolerability of a Solution Containing Propyl Betaine and Polihexanide for Wound Irrigation M. Romanelli V. Dini S. Barbanera M. S. Bertone Wound Healing Research Unit, Department of Dermatology, University of Pisa, Pisa, Italy *Skin Pharmacol Physiol* 2010;23(suppl 1):41–44 DOI: 10.1159/000318 266.

[35] Barbul A (2005) Wound healing. In: Brunicardi FC, Andersen DK, Billiar TR et al. (eds) *Schwartz's principles of surgery, Eighthth edn.* The McGraw-Hill Companies, Inc, Columbus, pp 165–182.

[36] Woo K, Ayello EA, Sibbald RG (2007) The edge effect: current therapeutic options to advance the wound edge. *Adv Skin Wound Care* 20(2):99–11.

[37] Percival NJ (2002) Classification of wounds and their management. *Surgery* 20(5):114–117.

[38] Howell JM, Chisholm CD (1992) Outpatient wound preparation and care: a national survey. *Ann Emerg Med* 21(8):976–981.

[39] Singer AJ, Hollander JE, Subramanian S, Malhotra AK, Villez PA (1994) Pressure dynamics of various irrigation techniques com- monly used in the emergency department. *Ann Emerg Med* 24 (1):36–40.

[40] Longmire AW, Broom LA, Burch J (1987) Wound infection following high-pressure syringe and needle irrigation. *Am J Emerg Med* 5(2):179–81.

[41] Rodeheaver GT, Ratliff (2008) Wound cleansing, wound irrigation, wound disinfection. In: Krasner D, Rodeheaver G, Sibbald RG (eds) Chronic wound care, Chapter 34. *HMP Communications*, Malvern.

[42] Hollander JE, Singer AJ, Valentine SM, Shofer FS (2001) Risk factors for infection in patients with traumatic lacerations. *Acad Emerg Med* 8(7):716–720.

[43] Chisholm CD, Cordell WH, Rogers K, Woods JR (1992) Comparison of a new pressurized saline canister versus syringe irrigation for laceration cleansing in the emergency department. *Ann Emerg Med* 21(11):1364–1367.

[44] Lammers RL, Hudson DL, Seaman ME (2003) Prediction of traumatic wound infection with a neural network-derived decision model. *Am J Emerg Med* 21(1):1–7.

[45] Grotz MR, Allami MK, Harwood P, Pape HC, Krettek C, Giannoudis PV (2005) Open pelvic fractures: epidemiology, current concepts of management and outcome. *Injury* 36(1):1–13.

[46] Fernandez R, Griffiths R (2008) Water for wound cleansing. *Cochrane Database Syst Rev* 23(1):CD003861.

[47] Khan MN, Naqvi AH (2006) Antiseptics, iodine, povidone iodine and traumatic wound cleansing. *J Tissue Viability* 16(4):6–10.

[48] Watt BE, Proudfoot AT, Vale JA (2004) Hydrogen peroxide poisoning. *Toxicol Rev* 23(1):51–57.

[49] Cartotto RC, Peters WJ, Neligan PC, Douglas LG, Beeston J (1996) Chemical burns. *Can J Surg* 39(3):205–211.

[50] Prucz RB, Sullivan SR, Klein MB. *Acute wound care. ACS surgery: principles and practice*. Ontario, Canada: Decker Intellectual Properties; 2012.

[51] Anglen JO. Wound irrigation in musculoskeletal injury. *J Am Acad Orthop Surg* 2001;9:219-26.

[52] Hays EP. Wound care: from door to discharge. *Proceedings of the Boston Scientific Assembly*; October 6, 2009; Boston, MA.

[53] Gabriel A, Schraga E, Windle ML. *Wound irrigation*. 2011. Available from: www.emedicine.medscape.com/article/1895071. Accessed July 20, 2013.

[54] Edmiston CE, Bruden B, Rucinski MC, Henen C, Graham MB, Lewis BL. Reducing the risk of surgical site infections: doeschlorhexidine gluconate provide a risk reduction benefit? *Am J Infect Control* 2013;41:549-55.

[55] Suzuki T, Sadahiro S, Maeda Y, Tanaka A, Okada K, Kamijo A. Optimal duration of prophylactic antibiotic administration for elective colon cancer surgery: A randomized, clinical trial. *Surgery.* 2011;149(2):171-8.

[56] Baas-Vrancken Peeters MJ, Kluit AB, Merkus JW, Breslau PJ. Short versus long-term postoperative drainage of the axilla after axillary lymph node dissection. A prospective randomized study. *Breast Cancer Res Treat.* 2005;93(3):271-5.

[57] *Global Guidelines for the Prevention of Surgical Site Infection.* I. World Health Organization. ISBN 978 92 4 154988 2 Subject headings are available from WHO institutional repository © World Health Organization 2016.

[58] Clegg-Lamptey JN, Dakubo JC, Hodasi WM. Comparison of four-day and ten-day post- mastectomy passive drainage in Accra, Ghana. *East Afr Med J.* 2007;84(12):561-5.

[59] Fernandez R, Griffiths R, Ussia C (2002) Water for wound cleansing. *Cochrane Database Syst Rev* 4, CD003861. doi:10.1002/14651858. cd003861.

[60] Cervantes-Sanchez CR, Gutierrez-Vega R, Vazquez-Carpizo JA, Clark P, Athie-Gutierrez C (2000) Syringe pressure irrigation of subdermic tissue after appendectomy to decrease the incidence of postoperative wound infection. *World J Surg* 24(1):38–41, discussion -2.

[61] Al-Ramahi M, Bata M, Sumreen I, Amr M (2006) Saline irrigation and wound infection in abdominal gynecologic surgery. *Int J Gynaecol Obstet* 94(1):33–36. doi:10.1016/j.ijgo.2006.03.030.

[62] Gungorduk K, Asicioglu O, Celikkol O, Ark C, Tekirdag AI (2010) Does saline irrigation reduce the wound infection in caesarean delivery? *J Obstet Gynaecol* 30(7):662–666. doi:10.3109/01443615.2010. 494206.

[63] Harrop JS, Styliaras JC, Ooi YC, Radcliff KE, Vaccaro AR, Wu C (2012) Contributing factors to surgical site infections. *J Am Acad Orthop Surg* 20(2):94–101. doi:10.5435/jaaos-20-02-094.

[64] Banwell H (2006) What is the evidence for tissue regeneration impairment when using a formulation of PVP-I antiseptic on open wounds? *Dermatology* 212(Suppl 1):66–76. doi:10.1159/000089202.

[65] Alexander JW, Solomkin JS, Edwards MJ (2011) Updated recommendations for control of surgical site infections. *Ann Surg* 253(6): 1082–1093. doi:10.1097/SLA.0b013e31821175f8.

[66] Tejwani NC, Immerman I (2008) Myths and legends in orthopaedic practice: are we all guilty? *Clin Orthop Relat Res* 466(11):2861–2872. doi:10.1007/s11999-008-0458-2.

[67] Alexander JW, Rahn R, Goodman HR (2009) Prevention of surgical site infections by an infusion of topical antibiotics in morbidly obese patients. *Surg Infect* 10(1):53–57. doi:10.1089/sur.2008.038.

[68] Whiteside OJ, Tytherleigh MG, Thrush S, et al. Intra- operative peritoneal lavage: Who does it and why? *Ann R Coll Surg Engl* 2005;87:255–258.

[69] BusinessWire. *Survey Conducted at AORN Congress Re- veals Need for New and Better Surgical Site Infection Prevention Strategies.* 2013 [Available at: www.businesswire.com/news/home/20130311 005412/en/Survey-Conducted-AORNCongress-Reveals-Surgical-Site.

[70] Galland RB, Saunders JH, Mosley JG, et al. Prevention of wound infection in abdominal operations by peroperative antibiotics or povidone–iodine: A controlled trial. *Lancet* 1977;2:1043–1045.

[71] Barnes S, Spencer M, Graham D, et al. Surgical wound irrigation: A call for evidence-based standardization of practice. *Am J Infect Control* 2014;42:525–529.

[72] Edmiston CE Jr, Bruden B, Rucinski MC, et al. Reducing the risk of surgical site infections: Does chlorhexidine gluconate provide a risk reduction benefit? *Am J Infect Control* 2013;41(5 Suppl):S49–S55.

[73] Edmiston CE Jr, Bruden B, Rucinski MC, et al. Reducing the risk of surgical site infections: Does chlorhexidine gluconate provide a risk reduction benefit? *Am J Infect Control* 2013;41:S49–S55.

[74] Platt J, Bucknall RA. An experimental evaluation of anti- septic wound irrigation. *J Hosp Infect* 1984;5:181–188.

[75] Reducing the risk of surgical site infections: Does chlorhexidine gluconate provide a risk reduction benefit? Charles E. Edmiston, Jr. PhD, *American Journal of Infection Control* 41 (2013) S49-S55.

[76] Centers for Disease Control and Prevention Guideline for the Prevention of Surgical Site Infection, 2017 Sandra I. Berríos-Torres, MD *JAMA Surg*. 2017;152(8):784-791. doi:10.1001/jamasurg.2017.0904 Published online May 3, 2017. Corrected on June 21, 2017.

[77] *WHO global guidelines for the prevention of surgical site infection.*

[78] Platell C, Papadimitriou JM, Hall JC. The influence of lavage on peritonitis. *J Am Coll Surg* 2000;191:672–80.

[79] Cervantes-Sanchez CR, Gutierrez-Vega R, Vasquez-Carpizio JA, et al. Syringe pressure ir- ritation of subdermic tissue after appendectomy to decrease the incidence of postoperative wound infection. *World J Surg* 2000;24:38–41.

[80] Andersen B, Bendtsen A, Holbraad L, et al. Wound infections after appendectomy. I. Acontrolled trial on the prophylactic efficacy of topical ampicillin in non-perforated appendicitis. *Acta Chir Scand* 1972;138:531–6.

[81] O'Connor LT Jr, Goldstein M. Topical perioperative antibiotic prophylaxis for minor clean inguinal surgery. *J Am Coll Surg* 2002; 194:407–10.

[82] The efficacy and risks of using povidone- iodine irrigation to prevent surgical site infection: an evidence-based review Josie Chundamala, MA; James G. Wright, MD, *MPH Can J Surg*, Vol. 50, No. 6, December 2007 473.

[83] Allegranzi B, ZayedB, Bischoff P, et al. New WHO recommendations in intraoperative and postoperative measures for surgical site infection prevention: an evidence-based global perspective. *Lancet Infect Dis* 2016;16:e288-e303.

[84] Costerton, JW, Stewart PS, Greenberg, EP: Bacterial biofilm: a common cause of persis- tent infections. *Science* 1999;284:1318–1322.

In: Prophylaxis of Surgical Site Infection … ISBN: 978-1-53615-615-7
Editors: Jaime Ruiz-Tovar et al. © 2019 Nova Science Publishers, Inc.

Chapter 10

TOPICAL INTRAPERITONEAL IRRIGATION

Jaime Ruiz-Tovar[1,], MD, PhD and Carolina Llavero[2,†]*

[1]Center of Excellence for the Study and Treatment of Obesity and Diabetes, Valladolid, Spain
[2]Department of Surgical Nursery, Sureste Hospital, Madrid, Spain

ABSTRACT

Peritoneal irrigation achieves a reduction in bacterial contamination. The addition of antibiotics has shown some benefits in experimental studies, but human ones have obtained controversial results. The evidence about the use of antiseptics is limited.

In this chapter we will review the available evidence.

Keywords: peritoneal irrigation, antibiotic, surgical-site infection

---

[*] Corresponding Author's Email: jruiztovar@gmail.com.
[†] Carolina Llavero, RN.

INTRODUCTION

Peritoneal lavage has been adopted by many surgeons for use in abdominal operations. This lavage usually consists of peritoneal irrigation with a variable volume of 0.9% sodium chloride (normal saline). The effects of lavage have been widely studied for management of patients with bacterial peritonitis, although the appropriate volume and carrier remain unclear, as does the benefit of including antibiotics or antiseptics. To reduce the morbidity and mortality of intraabdominal infections, surgeons aim to isolate and control the source of contamination. Lavage has been proposed to remove bacterial contamination and other materials that may promote bacterial proliferation (e.g., blood) and proinflammatory cytokines that may enhance local inflammation. Therefore, flushing the peritoneal cavity may reduce the bacterial load, inhibit bacterial proliferation, and possibly minimize peritoneal adhesions. Antibiotics may be combined with the lavage to further reduce bacterial survival. Antibiotics used have included metronidazole, gentamicin sulfate, cephalothin, lincomycin, kanamycin, doxycycline, and ampicillin. Nearly all of the previously reported studies were conducted in peritonitis situations, and most of them were under experimental conditions and stated that antibiotic lavage was safe. However, the efficacy of the lavage was not always demonstrated, especially when comparisons were made with historic controls.

Clearly, the efficacy of peritoneal irrigations in peritonitis is unclear. The concept of lavaging a contaminated or infected peritoneal cavity makes good sense intuitively. However, because microbes adhere to mesothelial cells, it is very difficult to wash them off the peritoneal surface. During fecal contamination of the peritoneal cavity, it has been demonstrated that bacteria that adhered to the mesothelium were resistant to intraperitoneal lavage, resulting in only transitory reductions of bacterial populations. Peritoneal irrigation with normal saline is not sufficient to eliminate all fecal contamination produced during the surgical act. The results obtained after antibiotic lavage defend the hypothesis that the topical effect of the antibiotics could completely inhibit the growth of bacteria in the peritoneum, even when microorganisms have adhered to the mesotelial cells. Diverse antimicrobial drugs have been used in different studies, most of which were peritonitis cases.

The results obtained are contradictory. Some authors have presented similar mortality and intra-abdominal infection rates compared with normal saline irrigation; others have shown antibiotic lavage to protect against intra-abdominal infection and reduce the mortality rate by up to 65%. A meta-analysis clearly shows the superior value of antibiotics in lavage during experimental peritonitis compared with saline lavage. Although including antibiotics in lavage solutions optimizes survival in peritonitis, the use of simple saline irrigation is still better than no lavage, rejecting the classical affirmation that irrigation contributes to contamination spread throughout the peritoneal cavity.

Peritoneal lavage with a single antibiotic drug is probably sufficient to impair the growth of some, but not all, bacterial colonies. Previous studies have not specified which microorganisms survived after antibiotic lavage. Logically, bacterial growth cannot be impaired by antibiotics to which the microorganisms are resistant.

Tolhurst Cleaver and colleagues reported that intraperitoneal antibiotic lavage accelerated wound healing and reduced the infection rate. Diverse factors contribute to the occurrence of wound infection, but infections arising from a contaminated peritoneal cavity are particularly common, indicating that wound infection rates are higher after a contaminated operation than after a clean one.

Qadan et al., noted that extrapolating results from animal models of peritonitis and antibiotic lavage to human disease is often disappointing, because in experimental peritonitis, the interval between the onset of peritonitis and the start of the lavage treatment is usually only 1 or 2 hours, which is not representative of the clinical situation (characterized by a longer time interval). A long interval between the onset of peritonitis and treatment leads to exponential growth of the microorganisms. In this situation, an antibiotic lavage would not be sufficient to control such concentrations of microorganisms but may be sufficient for lower concentrations of bacteria. Thus, peritoneal irrigation with antibiotic solutions has more sense as a prophylactic measure in elective surgery, rather than as treatment in peritoneal cases.

PROPHYLAXIS OF SSI WITH ANTIBIOTIC PERITONEAL IRRIGATION

In 2012, our group conducted a prospective randomized clinical trial, analyzing the peritoneal irrigation with normal saline (Group 1) vs the irrigation with a clincamycin-gentamicin solution (Group 2), on SSI after elective colorectal surgery. Inclusion criteria were a diagnosis of colorectal neoplasms and plans to undergo an elective operation with curative aims. An open surgical approach was used in all the patients included. Exclusion criteria were a preoperative diagnosis of chronic renal failure (because of the risk of nephrotoxicity associated with intraperitoneal gentamicin absorption) or an anastomotic leak in the postoperative course, which would represent a bias in the diagnosis of intra-abdominal infection. A CT scan with a rectal contrast enema was performed either on the fifth day after surgery or earlier if there was a strong clinical suspicion of an anastomotic leak. This procedure identified anastomotic leaks presenting as intra-abdominal abscesses rather than peritonitis.

Perioperative systemic antibiotics (ciprofloxacin 400 mg and metronidazol 1,500 mg; single dose preoperatively, within 30 minutes of incision, and redosed after 4 hours when the surgery is prolonged over that time) were used in both groups. No mechanical bowel preparation took place in any patient.

A total of 108 patients were included in the study. Five patients were excluded because they presented an anastomotic leak. In total, 51 patients were analyzed in Group 1 and 52 in Group 2. The patient sample consisted of 62% men and 38% women, with a mean age of 69.9 years. The preoperative diagnosis was adenocarcinoma in all patients. There were no differences in comorbidities and tumor stages between groups. Tumors were located in the right colon (17%), the transverse colon (3%), the left colon (50%), and the rectum (27%). In 3 patients, 2 synchronic neoplasms were detected in different locations of the colon. There were no significant differences in the surgical techniques between groups. Anastomosis was performed in 70% of the patients, leaving a terminal stoma in 30%. There were no significant differences in the distribution of patients with stomas between groups.

Anastomotic leaks appeared in 5 patients (5%), including 3 patients in Group 1 and 2 patients in Group 2 (nonsignificant, NS). Mortality was 3%, affecting 2 patients in Group 1 and 1 patient in Group 2 (NS). Causes of mortality were an anastomotic leak and sepsis in 2 patients and nosocomial pneumonia in 1 patient. Median hospital stays were 6 days (range 5 to 32 days) in Group 1 and 6.5 days (range 5 to 14 days) in Group 2 (NS).

The wound infection rates were 14% in Group 1 and 4% in Group 2 (p = 0.009; [odds ratio]OR4.94;95%CI 1.27 to 19.19). There was no significant association between any of the comorbidities and wound infection. Intraabdominal abscess rates were 6% in Group 1 and 0% in Group 2 (p = 0.014; OR 2.14; 95% CI 1.13 to 3.57). All abscesses were smaller than 4 cm and therefore were conservatively managed without requiring percutaneous drainage, so we could not obtain a sample of them for culture.

Microbiologic samples were obtained only from patients assigned to Group 2. The culture of sample 1 (before any lavage) was positive in 68% of the cases. Detected microorganisms were *Escherichia coli (E coli)* (94% of the samples),

Streptococcus spp (27%), *Enterococcus faecalis* (9%), *Pseudomonas aeruginosa* (6%), and *Klebsiella spp* (3%). The culture of sample 2 (after lavage with normal saline) was positive in 59% of the cases, and the same microorganisms identified in the culture of sample 1 were found in the culture of sample 2. The culture of sample 3 (after lavage with the antibiotic solution) was positive in 2 patients (4%). Detected microorganisms were *Klebsiella spp* and *Streptococcus salivarius*. The antibiogram of these microorganisms revealed that they were both resistant to gentamicin and clindamycin. There was no significant difference between the infection rates of samples 1 and 2 (p = 0.162). However, when comparing samples 1 and 3 and samples 2 and 3, a significant difference in the infection rate was observed (p = 0.001 in both cases).

The prophylactic effect of lavage in elective clean contaminated surgery is understood even less than in peritonitis because few such studies have been conducted, apart from our one. In our study, we showed that an antibiotic lavage is very effective. We demonstrated that an antibiotic lavage impairs microbiologic growth and reduced the positive culture. These data have clinical correlations because the intra-abdominal infection rate was reduced from 6% in Group 1 (only saline lavage) to 0% in Group 2 (saline lavage followed by antibiotic irrigation). Our study presents 2 main differences with the reported literature. First, our sample included patients undergoing elective colorectal surgery (contaminated surgery), but who did not present with peritonitis, as described in most reported studies. A limited number of outdated studies have analyzed the effect of prophylactic peritoneal lavage on postoperative infection. Such studies have shown a reduction in the number of aerobic and anaerobic bacteria in the peritoneal fluid after an intervention that included irrigation with a tetracycline solution, but they have not correlated these data with clinical variables. The second main difference in our study is the combination of antibiotic drugs (gentamicin and clindamycin). These 2 drugs present a synergistic effect and provide wide-spectrum protection against Gram-negative and anaerobic microorganisms, which represent the main flora of the colon.

In our study, we also observed a significant reduction in wound infections in the group undergoing an antibiotic lavage, compared with the group undergoing saline irrigation. These data show that when the peritoneal cavity remains sterile, there is a lower risk of bacteria migrating from the abdominal cavity through the fascia to the subcutaneous tissue. As in the 2 patients with positive cultures after antibiotic lavage, the same bacteria found in the culture were also responsible for the wound infection.

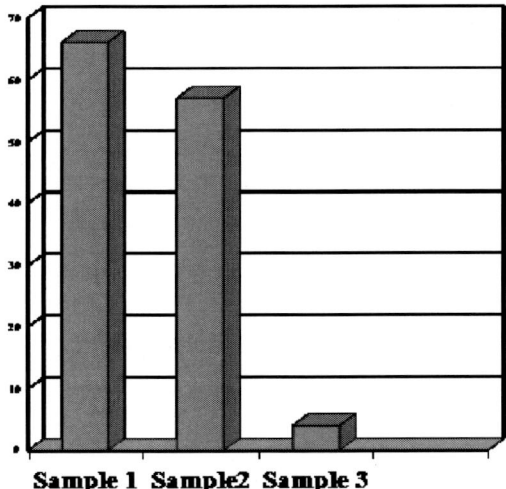

Figure 1. Peritoneal contamination before any lavage (Sample 1), after irrigation with normal saline (Sample 2) and after irrigation with antibiotic solution (Sample 3).

The conclusion of this study was that antibiotic lavage of the peritoneum before abdominal wall closure is associated with a lower incidence of intraabdominal abscesses and wound infection. Microbiologic cultures of the peritoneal surface at the end of an elective colorectal operation were positive in 68% of the cases. A normal saline lavage did not significantly reduce the number of positive cultures, in contrast to an antibiotic one (gentamicin-clindamycin), which resulted in negative cultures for all sensitive microorganisms. This study would support the use of antibiotical perritoneal irrigation as prophylactic measure against SSI. Moreover, the main criticism of the use of topical antibiotics is the development of eventual resistant microorganisms against the drugs used. In our opinion, the antibiotics used should be those ones not usually employed for treatment aims. In our study we used clindamycin, which is not a drug currently used for the treatment of intra-abdominal infections, and despite gentamicin is frequently used for the treatment of gramnegative infections, it is true that there are other more powerful aminoglucosides for treatment uses, and even gentamicin is included in many systemic prophylaxis protocols. Further studies must be conducted to confirm these hypotheses.

Topical Peritoneal Irrigation with Antiseptic Agents

Antiseptic agents, such as Polyvinylpirrolidone (Iodine Povidone) or Chlorhexidine have demonstrated an antibacterial effect and are currently used for topical antisepsia of skin or mucosae. However, the peritoneal surface has the characteristic of absorption and this limits the applicability of several drugs to this surface.

Experimental studies with peritoneal Povidone irrigation have demonstrated a significant reduction of SSI. Povidone irrigation reduces the permeability of the mesotelium to bacteria and, consequently might reduce the systemic spread of the microrganisms.

Studies on human have been conducted on patients with peritoneal carcinomatosis, aiming to reduce the tumoral load. However, this topical administration has shown a certain peritoneal absorption and may lead to systemic toxicity. Moreover, several patients developed sclering peritonitis. Thus, peritoneal Povidone administration is actually not recommended.

Periotneal irrigation with Chlorehexidine has also demonstrated in experimental studies a significant reduction of bacterial contamination. However, an important chemical irritation was also observed, leading to extense inflammatory response. Long-term follow-up of these patients has shown the development of peritoneal adhesion and bowel obstruction. However, the latter has not been confirmed in recent animal studies. Thus, the role of topical Chlorhexidine in peritoneal irrigations must be further elucidated.

CONCLUSION

Peritoneal irrigation achieves a reduction in bacterial contamination. The addition of antibiotics has shown some benefits as prophylactic measure against SSI. However, there is still no enough evidence to be a recommended measure by scientific societies. Povidone and Chlorhexidine solutions seems to be associated with greater adverse events than benefits and are actually not recommended for peritoneal irrigation.

REFERENCES

Adam U, Ledwon D, Hopt UT. Programmed lavage as a basic principle in therapy of diffuse peritonitis. *Langenbecks Arch Surg* 1997;382:18–21.

Araujo ID, Grossi GC, Diniz SO, et al. Effects of the povidone-iodine (PVPI) in treatment of bacterial peritonitis induced in rats. *Acta Cir Bras* 2010; 25:322-327.

Edmiston CE Jr, GoheenMP, Kornhall S, et al. Fecal peritonitis: microbial adherence to serosal mesothelium and resistance to peritoneal lavage. *World J Surg* 1990;14:176–183.

Grant SW, Hopkins J, Wilson SE. Operative site bacteriology as an indicator of postoperative infectious complications in elective colorectal surgery. *Am Surg* 1995;61:856–861.

Hall JC, Heel KA, Papadimitriou J, Platell C. The pathobiology of peritonitis. *Gastroenterology* 1998;114:185–196.

Horiuchi T, Tanishima H, Tamagawa K, et al. A wound protector shields incision sites from bacterial invasion. *Surg Infect (Larchmt)* 2010;11:501–503.

Parc Y, Frileux P, Schmitt G, et al. Management of postoperative peritonitis after anterior resection: experience from a referral intensive care unit. *Dis Colon Rectum* 2000;43:579–587.

Platell C, Papadimitriou JM, Hall JC. The influence of lavage on peritonitis. *J Am Coll Surg* 2000;191:672–680.

Qadan M, Dajani D, Dickinson A, Polk HC. Meta-analysis of the effect of peritoneal lavage on survival in experimental peritonitis. *Br J Surg* 2010;97:151–159.

Ruiz-Tovar J, Santos J, Arroyo A, et al. Effect of Peritoneal Lavage with Clindamycin-Gentamicin Solution on Infections after Elective Colorectal Cancer Surgery. *J Am Coll Surg* 2012;214:202-207.

Saha SK. Efficacy of metronidazole lavage in treatment of intraperitoneal sepsis. A prospective study. *Dig Dis Sci* 1996;41: 1313–1318.

Shams WE, Hanley GA, Orvik A, et al. Peritoneal lavage using chlorhexidine gluconate at the end of colon surgery reduces postoperative intra-abdominal infection in mice. *J Surg Res* 2015; 195:121-127.

Silverman SH, Ambrose NS, Youngs DJ, et al. The effect of peritoneal lavage with tetracycline solution on postoperative infection. A prospective, randomized, clinical trial. *Dis Colon Rectum* 1986;29:165–169.

Sortini D, Feo CV, Maravegias K, et al. Role of peritoneal lavage in adhesion formation an survival rate in rats: an experimental study. *J Invest Surg* 2006;19:291–297.

Thoroughman J, Alker l, Collins J. Spreading organisms by peritoneal lavage. *Am J Surg* 1968;115:339–340.

Tolhurst Cleaver CL, Hopkins AD, Kee Kwong KC, Raftery AT. The effect of postoperative peritoneal lavage on survival, wound healing and adhesion formation following fecal peritonitis: an experimental study in the rat. *Br J Surg* 1974;61: 601–604.

In: Prophylaxis of Surgical Site Infection … ISBN: 978-1-53615-615-7
Editors: Jaime Ruiz-Tovar et al. © 2019 Nova Science Publishers, Inc.

Chapter 11

PROPHYLACTIC VACUUM THERAPY

Montiel Jiménez-Fuertes[*], *MD, PhD*
General and Digestive Surgery,
Rey Juan Carlos University Hospital, Madrid, Spain

ABSTRACT

Surgical site infections are an important complication after surgery, affecting the quality of life and the economic cost. It is important to note that infections are multifactorial, involving both surgical and patient factors. To decrease the occurrence of infections, surgeons frequently use several tools to reduce the incidence of them. Strategies that prevent surgical site infection (SSI) are increasingly important and current literature suggests that incisional Negative Pressure Wound Therapy (iNWPT) is a promising intervention.

Keywords: negative pressure wound therapy, prophylaxis, incision management, surgical-site infection

---

[*] Corresponding Author's Email: montiel.jimenez@hospitalreyjuancarlos.es.

INTRODUCTION

Surgical site infections (SSI) are the most common cause of nosocomial infection, because they are the 38% of all hospital-acquired infections. Though the overall incidence of SSI is low, the highest rates occur after abdominal surgery [1].

Surgical site infections (SSI) are categorized as superficial incisional, deep incisional, and organ/space based on the depth of the infection, they can increase healthcare costs by approximately $20,000 per admission, and add an average of 10 days of length-of-stay [2]. Given this effect on patient outcomes and costs, much work has been done to develop interventions that can decrease the rate of SSI. The most data have been produced in the fields of colorectal, gynecology, and urology which involve manipulation of the gastrointestinal or genitourinary systems; or in fields in which placement of prostheses require all effort to reduce SSI, such as orthopedics, neurosurgery and cardiothoracic. There have been many skin closure adjuncts employed to reduce SSI, pre-closure, wound irrigation, and some are post-closure such as topical antibiotic agents and incisional negative pressure wound treatment (iNPWT) applied to a closed incision. All, however, remain debatable as to their efficacy despite having been studied in many surgical settings.

Incisional Negative Pressure Wound Treatment

Incisional negative pressure wound treatment (iNPWT) has emerged as a useful tool to reduce surgical site infections (SSIs) [3]. INPWT technology has been developed like Prevena™ (KCI USA, Inc., San Antonio, TX) and Pico (Smith & Nephew Inc, Andover, MA) systems. Both have been created to develop prophylactic measures to prevent complications via application immediately after surgery in high-risk closed surgical incisions. NPWT involves the controlled application of continuous sub-atmospheric pressure to the wound. While NPWT technology is an established and accepted treatment for non-healing wounds and open surgical incisions following infection, a small but growing number of clinical studies have been published based on the hypothesis that negative pressure dressings improve healing of closed wounds.

Prevena™ Incision Management system consists of a vacuum therapy suction unit that is connected to a dressing tube by a canister for fluid collection, and a precut peel-and-place reticulated open-cell foam dressing specifically designed for use over closed surgical incisions that are at high risk for post-surgical complications (*Figures 1 and 2*). The dressing has a plated non-adherent layer surrounding the foam and a semi-permeable adhesive drape.

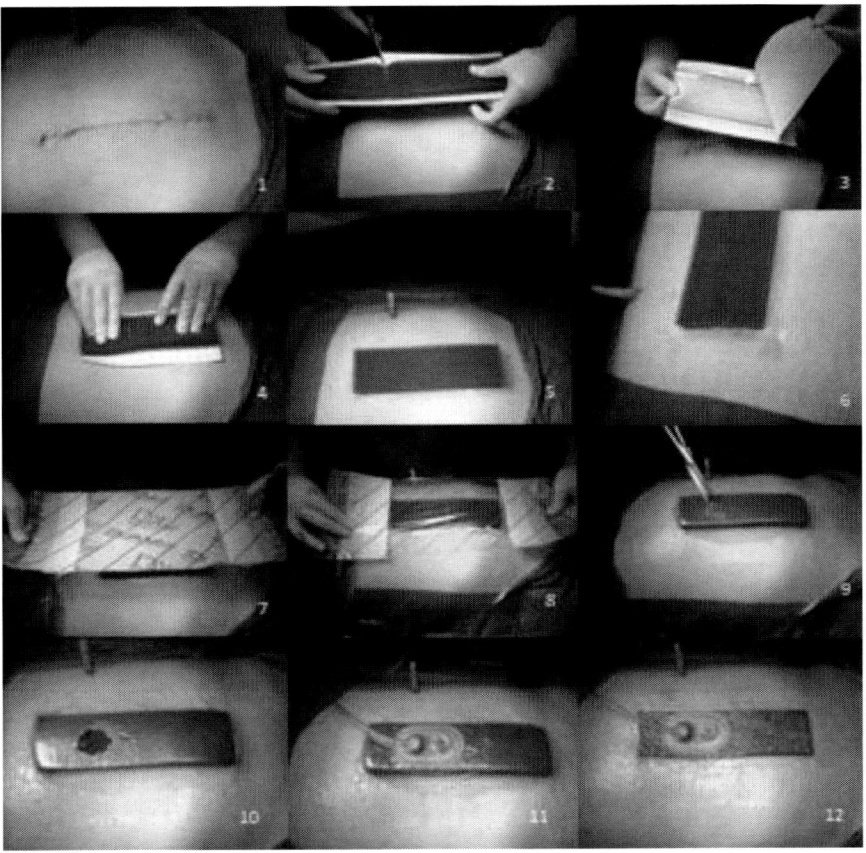

Figure 1. Prevena™ Incision Management system: 1: closed wound; 2-11: customizable prevena placemet step by step; 12: final view with de dressing working.

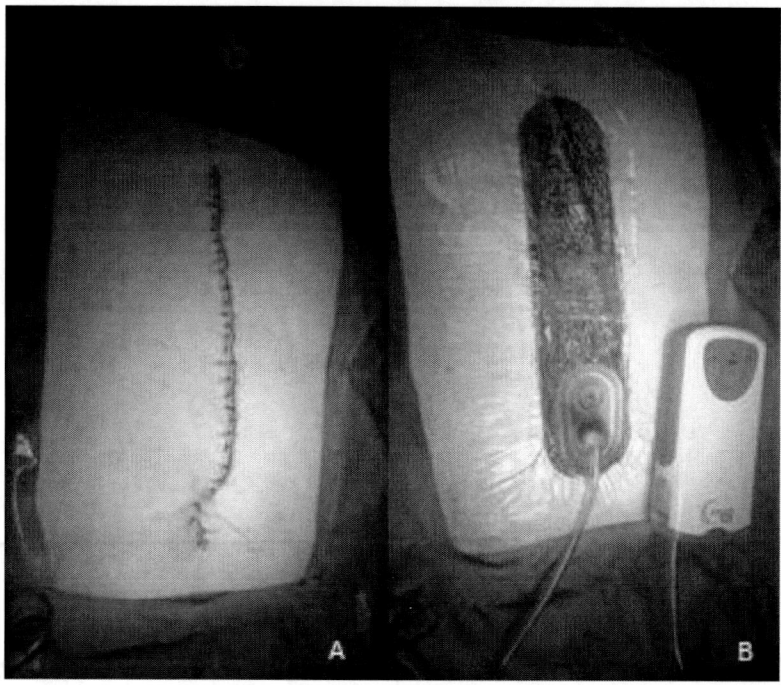

Figure 2. Prevena™ Incision Management system. A: Abdominal closed wound; B: Prevena™ in place and working.

Pico systems is canister-free, the pump generates a negative pressure of − 80 mmHg (for 7 days of therapy) and is connected to a dressing that manages the fluid away from the wound or closed incision through a unique combination of absorbency and evaporation.

An increased understanding of the science behind incisional NPWT and its effects on wound and periwound tissue is essential to expand the use of incisional NPWT. Well-described mechanisms of action of incisional NPWT include protection of the incision site from external infectious sources and help in holding incision edges together [4]. Incisional NPWT also removes fluids and infectious materials from the surgical site, which is especially important in critical anatomical locations. Other mechanisms of action, particularly at the cellular and molecular level, are less understood and the subject of ongoing research [5].

EFFECTS OF INCISIONAL NEGATIVE WOUND PRESSURE DRESSING IN WOUNDS

Surgical incisions disrupt the cutaneous layer that normally doesn't let bacteria entering the body. In healthy people it takes three to six days for reepithelialization to restore the barrier function of the skin. Risk factors such as diabetes or contaminated surgical fields such as related to abdominal surgical procedures with intestinal anastomoses result in prolonged time to healing [6]. Post-operative colonization of surgical sites is associated with increased risk of SSI [7].

NPWT's ways to prevent SSIs includes completely eliminating dead space, removing fluid and blood, improving blood flow and preventing the formation of subcutaneous seromas/hematomas that become secondarily infected. In addition, INPWT is thought to decrease local inflammatory response and cell death by increasing the oxygen gradient across a wound.

The NPWT dressing is applied to the surgical site under sterile conditions, after which a continuous amount of sub-atmospheric pressure is applied for several post-operative days. Most studies report use of - 80 or - 125mm Hg of sub-atmospheric pressure, for a length of five to seven days after operation.

Jansen et al. [5] demostrated a correlation between external negative pressure applied by the iNPWT system and the pressure within the wound. Even low external negative pressure (about 50 mmHg) led to relevant negative pressure within the wound.

Barrier Function of NPWT

Because of its non-occlusive nature, gauze and other dressings are permeable to bacteria [8]. Lawrence et al. [9] have demonstrated that bacteria can pass through up to 64 layers of dry gauze in a *in vitro* study. In contrast, iNPWT uses a foil that is impermeable to pathogens. INPWT devices have the ability of the dressing to serve as a barrier against external contamination, and this was verified through a Phi-X 174 bacteriophage challenge. This test indicated that there was no pathogenpenetration through the foil [10]. Moreover, the subatmospheric pressure results in close approximation of the foil to several centimeters of skin, while also approximating both incisional edges. Anything that passes through the incision is also directed away from the surgical site as a result of the direction of suction, and in this way it acts as a barrier against external bacteria. This is in line with the clinical results of Grauhan et al. [11], who have found that iNPWT resulted in a significant reduction of SSI from (grampositive) skin flora after cardiac surgical procedures in obese individuals (1/75 vs. 10/75, $p = 0.009$). Moreover, because an iNPWT dressing commonly is left in place for 7 days, less dressing changes [12] and bedside examinations take place, and by decreasing the exposure of the surgical site to potential colonization from the nurses.

Seroma, Hematoma and Edema Reduction

Seroma development is one of the most commonly reported complication, and both are associated with an increased risk of SSI [13]. Hematomas and seromas result from the accumulation of blood and serum, respectively, in internal spaces. Even with an excellent surgical technique, bleeding, inflammation and serum extravasation may occur, resulting in increased probability of infection, slower healing, additional clinic visits and surgical re-interventions.

In vivo studies have provided evidence of improved fluid flow with four days of continuous INPWT (Prevena™ Incision Dressing) under −125 mmHg over clean, closed incisions, showing that its application, when compared with semi-permeable film dressing (Tegaderm™ Dressing, St. Paul, MN, USA), significantly decreased the amount of porcine subcutaneous dead spaces beneath superficial closed incisions indicating reduced haematoma/seroma [14]. In humans, there are several randomized controlled trials, of wich several reported decreased seroma and hematoma formation, but there are others that didn't see this effect [15-19].

Edema has a detrimental effect in wound healing because of the increased diffusion distance for oxygen, and the oxygen is important for bacterial clerance [20]. It has been suggested that iNPWT is effective at reducing edema, which increases tissue oxygenation and thereby bacterial clearance [21].

Effect of iNPWT on Perfusion and Necrosis

A good perfusion and oxygenation are essential for a good surgical site healing. In the first animal study on NPWT, Morykwas et al. [22] have shown that the cutaneous application of NPWT onto ischemic skin flaps made a significant reduction of cutaneous necrosis in their porcine model. Correspondingly, cutaneous application of NPWT results in a perfusion increase when applied to intact skin of healthy volunteers [23], and in significantly increased perfusion at post-operative days four, seven, and 21, as measured with laser Doppler perfusion imaging [24-25].

Wound Dehiscence

The biomechanic effects of iNWPT on closed wounds have been evaluated with computer models and they showed that iNPWT reduces the lateral distraction force in wounds [26], and this is important because a wound dehiscence increases the risk or SSI due to bacteria contamination.

SSI

INPWT seems to be effective in the prevention of SSI acting as a barrier which avoids bacteria contamination of the wound before healing, improving the lymphatic and bood flow, reducing seroma, hematoma, edema and wound dehiscence. This suggests that iNPWT is a favorable prevention strategy to consider. This is substantiated in part by the clinical data available, as assessed in meta-analyses that show that iNPWT reduces SSI [1]. This suggests that iNPWT is effective in reducing the risk of SSI in all types of surgical procedures, and likely even in the types of operations where no clinical data exist yet. Because of these results, the World Health Organization recommends to consider iNPWT for all highrisk surgical sites [27].

Conclusion

INPWT is an effective intervention as the result of its barrier function and optimization of the wound microenvironment. Incorporation of iNPWT in SSI prevention bundles is recommended supported by the data available in this moment.

References

[1] Zwanenburg, PR; Tol, BT; de Vries, FEE; Boermeester, MA. Incisional Negative Pressure Wound Therapy for Surgical Site Infection Prophylaxis in the Post-Antibiotic Era. *Surg Infect (Larchmt).*, 2018, Sep 29 [Epub ahead of print].

[2] Lawrence, SA; McIntyre, CA; Pulvirenti, A; Seier, K; Chou, Y; Gonen, M; et al. Perioperative Bundle to Reduce Surgical Site Infection after Pancreaticoduodenectomy: A Prospective Cohort Study. *J Am Coll Surg.*, 2019, Jan 7.

[3] Scalise, A; Calamita, R; Tartaglione, C; Pierangeli, M; Bolletta, E; Gioacchini, M; et al. Improving wound healing and preventing surgical site complications of closed surgical incisions: a possible role of Incisional Negative Pressure Wound Therapy. A systematic reviewof the literature. *International Wound Journal*, 2016, 1260–1281.

[4] Wilkes, RP; Kilpad, DV; Zhao, Y; Kazala, R; McNulty, A. Closed incision management with negative pressure wound therapy (CIM): biomechanics. *Surg Innov.*, 2012, 19, 67-75.

[5] Jansen-Winkeln, B; Niebisch, S; Scheuermann, U; Gockel, I; Mehdorn, M. Biomechanical Effects of Incisional Negative Wound Pressure Dressing: An *Ex Vivo* Model Using Human and Porcine Abdominal Walls. *Biomed Res Int.*, 2018, 7058461.

[6] Streubel, PN; Stinner, DJ; Obremskey, WT. Use of negative-pressure wound therapy in orthopaedic trauma. *J Am Acad OrthopSurg*, 2012, 20(9), 564-574.

[7] Turtiainen, J; Hakala, T; Hakkarainen, T; Karhukorpi, J. The impact of surgical wound bacterial colonization on the incidence of surgical site infection after lower limb vascular surgery: A prospective observational study. *Eur J Vasc Endovasc Surg*, 2014, 47, 411–417.

[8] Sood, A; Granick, MS; Tomaselli, NL. Wound dressings and comparative effectiveness data. *Adv Wound Care (New Rochelle)*, 2014, 3, 511–529.

[9] Lawrence, JC. Dressings and wound infection. *Am J Surg*, 1994, 167, 21S–24S.

[10] *FDA. PREVENA_ Incision Management System 510(k) Premarket Notification.*, 2010. www.accessdata.fda.gov/ cdrh_docs/pdf10/ K100821.pdf.

[11] Grauhan, O; Navasardyan, A; Hofmann, M; Müller, P; Stein, J; Hetzer, R. Prevention of poststernotomy wound infections in obese patients by negative pressure wound therapy. *J Thorac Cardiovasc Surg*, 2013, 145, 1387–1392.

[12] Nherera, LM; Trueman, P; Karlakki, SL. Cost-effectiveness analysis of single-use negative pressure wound therapy dressings (sNPWT) to reduce surgical site complications (SSC) in routine primary hip and knee replacements. *Wound Repair Regen*, 2017, 25, 474–482.

[13] Vieira, BL; Qin, CD; Jordan, SW; Gutowski, KA; Kim, J. Assessing the association between seroma and surgical site infection in immediate breast reconstruction. *Plast Reconstr Surg Glob Open*, 2016, 4, (Suppl 9), p. 170.

[14] Kilpadi, DV; Cunningham, MR. Evaluation of closed incision management with negative pressure wound therapy (CIM): hematoma/seroma and involvement of the lymphatic system. *Wound Repair Regen*, 2011, 19, 588–96.

[15] Hyldig, N; Birke-Sorensen, H; Kruse, M; Vinter, C; Joergensen, JS; Sorensen, JA; et al. Metaanalysis of negative-pressure wound therapy for closed surgical incisions. *Br J Surg*, 2016, 103, 477–486.

[16] Angspatt, A; Laopiyasakul, T; Pungrasmi, P; Suwajo, P. The role of negative-pressure wound therapy in latissimus dorsi flap donor site seroma prevention: A cohort study. *Arch Plast Surg*, 2017, 44, 308–312.

[17] de Vries, FE; Atema, JJ; Lapid, O; Obdeijn, MC; Boermeester, MA. Closed incision prophylactic negative pressure wound therapy in patients undergoing major complex abdominal wall repair. *Hernia*, 2017, 2, 583–589.

[18] Redfern, RE; Cameron-Ruetz, C; O'Drobinak, SK; Chen, JT; Beer, KJ. Closed incision negative pressure therapy effects on postoperative infection and surgical site complication after total hip and knee arthroplasty. *J Arthroplasty*, 2017, 32, 3333–3339.

[19] Nickl, S; Steindl, J; Langthaler, D; et al. First experiences with incisional negative pressure wound therapy in a highrisk poststernotomy patient population treated with pectoralis major muscle flap for deep sternal wound infection. *J Reconstr Microsurg*, 2018, 34, 1–7.

[20] Knighton, DR; Fiegel, VD; Halverson, T; Schneider, S; Brown, T; Wells, CL. Oxygen as an antibiotic. The effect of inspired oxygen on bacterial clearance. *Arch Surg*, 1990, 125, 97–100.

[21] Perry, KL; Rutherford, L; Sajik, DM; Bruce, M. A preliminary study of the effect of closed incision management with negative pressure wound therapy over high-risk incisions. *BMC Vet Res*, 2015, 11, 279.

[22] Morykwas, MJ; Argenta, LC; Shelton-Brown, EI; McGuirt, W. Vacuum-assisted closure: A new method for wound control and treatment: Animal studies and basic foundation. *Ann Plast Surg*, 1997, 38, 553–562.

[23] Timmers, MS; Le Cessie, S; Banwell, P; Jukema, GN. The effects of varying degrees of pressure delivered by negative-pressure wound therapy on skin perfusion. *Ann Plast Surg*, 2005, 55, 665–671.

[24] Atkins, BZ; Tetterton, JK; Petersen, RP; Hurley, K; Wolfe, WG. Laser Doppler flowmetry assessment of peristernal perfusion after cardiac surgery: Beneficial effect of negative pressure therapy. *Int Wound J*, 2011, 8, 56–62.

[25] Peter Suh, HS; Hong, JP. Effects of incisional negativepressure wound therapy on primary closed defects after superficial circumflex iliac artery perforator flap harvest: Randomized controlled study. *Plast Reconstr Surg*, 2016, 138, 1333–1340.

[26] Loveluck, J; Copeland, T; Hill, J; Hunt, A; Martin, R. Biomechanical modeling of the forces applied to closed incisions during single-use negative pressure wound therapy. *Eplasty*, 2016, 16, e20.

[27] Allegranzi, B; Zayed, B; Bischoff, P; Kubilay, NZ; Zayed, B; Gomes, SM; et al. New WHO recommendations on intraoperative and postoperative measures for surgical site infection prevention: An evidence-based global perspective. *Lancet Infect Dis*, 2016, 16, e288–e303.

In: Prophylaxis of Surgical Site Infection … ISBN: 978-1-53615-615-7
Editors: Jaime Ruiz-Tovar et al. © 2019 Nova Science Publishers, Inc.

Chapter 12

ANTIMICROBIAL SUTURES

Jaime Ruiz-Tovar[1], MD, PhD and Carolina Llavero[*,2]

[1]Center of Excellence for the Study and Treatment of Obesity
and Diabetes, Valladolid, Spain
[2]Department of Surgical Nursery, Sureste Hospital, Madrid, Spain

ABSTRACT

The suture used for the aponeurotical closure might influence in the incidence of surgical-site infection (SSI). Microrganisms adhere to the suture material, specially in multifilament ones, and can show a relevant proliferation far away from the action of prophylactic systemic antibiotics. The use of sutures embebbed with antiseptic agents has demonstrated to reduce the incidence of incisional SSI.

The aim of this chapter is to review the actual evidence about this issue and to show the most relevant recommendations of several scientific societies.

Keywords: antimicrobial sutures, triclosan-coated sutures, surgical site infection

---

[*] Carolina Llavero, RN.

INTRODUCTION

Surgical-site infection (SSI) is one of the most frequent complications of abdominal surgery. It is associated with prolonged hospital stay, reduction of quality of life and increases of morbidity, mortality and sanitary costs. The reported incidence of SSI depends, among other factors, on the definition of SSI. The Centers for Disease Control (CDC) define SSI as the infection appearing in the surgical incision or close to it, during the first 30 days after surgery, or up to 3 months postoperatively, when a prosthesis has been placed. SSI occurs when the bacterial inoculum overcomes the ability of the immune system to control it. The bacterial contamination in abdominal surgery comes from the skin and the target organs during the surgical intervention.

The determinants of infection are the surgeon, the pathogen and the patient. The surgeon is the main modulator of surgical infection. Its experience and ability might reduce the inoculum to small dimensions, amenable to be controlled by the host defenses. A correct surgical act comprises a careful management of the tissues, a correct hemostasis, to avoid unnecessary prolongations of the surgical act and to minimize the exit of intraluminal content. Factors depending on the patient include comorbidities, obesity, tobacco habit and elderly. During the last decades, the pattern of microrganisms causing the infection has not changed, but the rate of resistant microrganisms.

The surgeon has pharmacological and non-pharmacological measures to reduce bacterial contamination from the surgical field and consequently the incidence of SSI. During the las decade, the use of bundles has become popular, as groups of systematic measures used for the prevention of postoperative complications. These bundles have been especially popular in colorectal surgery, which are considered high-risk procedures for infectious complications. In 2004, the CDC began the *Surgical Infection Prevention Project* (SIP), to assure the follow-up of several basic evidence-based measures for SSI prevention (adequate use of antibiotic prophylaxis, its administration 1h before skin incision and stop before 24h after surgery, appropriate hair removal and maintenance of normotermia). When applying these measures, Hendrick et al. reported in 2007 a better implementation of the prophylaxis protocol and a SSI reduction from 25.6% to 15.9% in colorectal surgery. However, a similar study did not confirm these findings, despite an improvement in all the aspects of the prophylaxis process. In 2011, a randomized study of 211 colorectal surgeries compared the implementation of a classic bundle with a bundle including, avoidance of mechanical colon preparation and oral antibiotic administration. Despite improvements in the implementations were observed, an increase in SSI rate from 24% to 45% was detected. In Spain, a multicentric observational study, analyzing the incidence of SSI in colorectal surgery, with implementation of a bundle similar to that from the SIP project, obtained a SSI rate of 23.1% in 611 colorectal interventions.

In conclusion, the adoption of bundles of evidence-based preventive measures against SSI lead to an improvement in the surgical process. The adhesion to the bundles by means of a check-list has shown to reduce SSI rates. However, there are still unknown factors implied in the development of SSI, that must be further investigated.

SUTURES EMBEBBED WITH ANTISEPTIC AGENTS

The use of sutures coated or embebbed with antiseptics are preventive measures against SSI, that can be implemented by the surgeon. Several studies has demonstrated that the suture used for the aponeurotical closure is a relevant factor that might influence the incidence of SSI. Bacteria adhere to the filaments of the suture, especially in multifilament ones. Thus, monofilament sutures are widely recommended for fascial closures, as with these sutures there is a lower place for bacterial accommodation.

In abdominal surgery, bacterial contamination comes from the digestive tract (*Enterobacteriacea* and anaerobic microrganisms) and from the saprophytic flora of the skin (grampositive). Sutures coated with antiseptic agents were designed to form a barrier against the bacterial transit from the intraperitoneal cavity to the subcutaneous tissue, that might lead to the development of incisional SSI. Moreover, their bactericide effect would prevent from bacterial adhesion to the suture filaments.

The most employed antiseptic agent used to coat the sutures is Triclosan (2,4,4-trichloro-2-hydroxi-diphenileter). In preclinical studies, Triclosan has demonstrated to reduce the bacterial load in the wound and to slow bacterial growth, inhibiting the synthesis of bacterial fatty acids.

Triclosan-coated sutures have been analyzed in different surgical procedures in humans, though most of them were conducted in clean and clean-contaminated ones. Among them, colorectal surgery has been the most widely procedure investigated, as the high incisional SSI rates that present, make these approaches as the most amenable to perform investigations on them. However, Triclosan-coated sutures have also demonstrated their efficacy in dirty surgery. A previous study of our group evaluated the efficacy of Triclosan-coated sutures in fecal peritonitis, revealing that the use of these sutures might reduce the incidence of incisional SSI in up to 80%.

Evidence

Up to date, 10 meta-analyses have been published, evaluating the efficacy of Triclosan-coates sutures, demonstrating all of the a reduction in SSI rates, ranging from 24% to 84%.

Wang et al. were the first who published a systematic review and meta-analysis on Triclosan-coated sutures in 2013. They included 17 clinical trials and 3720 patients were enrolled. Triclosan-coated sutures showed a 30% reduction of SSI. Subgroup analyses revealed homogeneous results in adults, abdominal procedures, and clean and clean-contaminated procedures.

The same year, Sajid et al. conducted a systematic review of clinical trials evaluating the effect of antibacterial sutures on skin closure. Seven studies with 1631 patients were included. They concluded that Triclosan-coated sutures reduced the SSI rate, but a significant reduction of hospital stay could not be observed.

Edmiston et al. performed a systematic review of 13 clinical trials with 3668 patients, showing that the use of antibacterial sutures was associated with a 31% global reduction of SSI, but it can reach up to 47% in selected populations.

The same authors published the next year a new systematic revision, including more rigorous methodology and updated the results with 2 additional clinical trials (totally 15 clinical trials and 4800 patients). They concluded that the use of Triclosan-coated sutures reduced the SSI risk in 33%. Depending on the degree of contamination, they observed that the risk reduction was applicable to clean, clean-contaminated and contaminated procedures, with evidence grade 1A.

In 2015, Apisarnthanarak et al. published a systematic review, including 22 clinical trials and 7 non-randomized studies. A 26% reduction of SSI risk ewas observed among clinical trials and a 47% reduction among non-randomized studies. In abdominal surgeries a 44% reduction was determined.

Guo et al. published in 2013 a meta-analysis of 13 clinical trials with 5256 participants. They performed a subgroup analysis based on the type of suture (Polyglactine 910 or Polydioxanone), coated or not with Triclosan. Globally, coated sutures were associated with a 24% lower risk of SSI. Depending on the type of surgery, the SSI risk was reduced a 30% in abdominal surgery within the patients undergoing Triclosan-coated sutures, but significant differences were not established in cardiac, mammary or other extra-abdominal procedures. The beneficial effect was determined both with the use of Triclosan-coated Polyglactine or Polydioxanone sutures, when compared with their corresponding Triclosan-free sutures. SSI reduction was associated with reduction of hospital stay and sanitary costs.

In 2017, Wu et al. performed a meta-regression analysis to determine if the effect of Triclosan varies depending on the type of suture or procedure. They included 13 clinical trials and 5 observational studies. Triclosan-coated sutures presented a 28% lower SSI rate among clinical trials and 42% lower risk among observational studies. The effect of the Triclosan coat was similar in the different types of sutures and procedures. The quality of evidence was moderate.

De Jonge published a 39% reduction of SSI risk with the use of Triclosan-coated sutures, after analyzing 21 clinical trials and 6462 patients.

Leaper et al. analyzed the clinical and economic impact of the use of these sutures. They analyzed 34 studies. Despite the incisional SSI rate was lower with the use of Triclosan coated sutures, the reduction was more pronounced in contaminated and dirty procedures. A 39% SSI reduction was estimated implying a mean sanitary cost reduction of 105€ per procedures among all types of surgeries, with 65€ reduction in clean surgeries and 285€ in contaminated or dirty ones.

In contrast, the meta-analysis of Konstantelias et al., including 30 studies, 19 of the clinical trials, and more than 15000 patients, observed that the use of Triclosan-coated sutures was associated with lower SSI risk in clean, clean-contaminated and contaminated procedures, but not in dirty ones. Especifically in colorectal surgery, they determined a reduction of 42% in the risk of SSI development. Moreover, a lower risk of wound dehiscence was also observed.

RECOMMENDATIONS OF SCIENTIFIC SOCIETIES

Based on all this scientific evidence, diverse organizations and societies have published recommendations, supporting the use of Triclosan-coated sutures.

World Health Organization (WHO)

In the paragraph 4.22 of the WHO recommendations for SSI prevention, the panel of experts recommend the use of Triclosan-coated sutures to reduce SSI, independently of the type of surgery. Evidence was cataloged as moderate. The effect seems to be independent from the type of suture (monofilament or multifilament), surgical procedure and wound contamination.

To establish this recommendation, 13 clinical trials and 5 observational studies were analyzed, including more than 7400 patients, comparing Triclosan-coated vs conventional sutures. The recommendation established by the WHO is considered conditional, as coated sutures are more expensive and their avalilability is limited in many countries. However, the uses of Triclosan-coated sutures might reduce mean hospital stay and, consequently, sanitary costs. They mentioned the possibility of development of resistances as a worrisome issue, but the daily absorption of Triclosan in many products, such as hand soap, is superior to that associated to a Triclosan-coated suture.

Centers for Disease Control and Prevention (CDC)

In the paragraph 2C, within the non-parenteral antimicrobial prophylactic measures, the use of Triclosan-coated sutures is included (Category II, low recommendation grade, moderate evidence). The evidence suggests that benefits compense prejudices. No benefit was observed for the prevention of organ/space SSI.

This recommendation was based on the analysis of 14 randomized controlled studies, including 5388 patients.

There is no evidence of antimicrobial resistances, adverse events or wound dehiscence.

American College of Surgeons and Surgical Site Infection Society

Historically, Triclosan-coated sutures were not recommended for SSI prevention, but actually there is enough evidence to support their use. Diverse studies have demonstrated a lower risk of SSI development with their use, when compared with standard sutures, including multiple clinical trials. Additionally, systematic reviews and meta-analysis have confirmed this effect.

Thus, these societies recommend the use of antibacterial sutures, but with 2 conditions:

- They must be used exclusively for the suture of aponeurotic layers, subcutaneous tissue and skin in abdominal surgeries, but their use is not justified for visceral sutures.
- The contamination grade must be clean or clean-contaminated. There is no enough evidence to justify their use in contaminated or dirty procedures.

REFERENCES

Allegranzi, B; Zayed, B; Bischoff, P; et al. New WHO recommendations on intraoperative and postoperative measures for surgical site infection prevention: an evidence-based global perspective. *Lancet Infect Dis.*, 2016, 16, e288-e303.

Anthony, T; Long, J; Hynan, LS; Sarosi, Jr. GA; Nwariaku, F; Huth, J; et al. Surgical complications exert a lasting effect on disease-specific health-related quality of life for patients with colorectal cancer. *Surgery.*, 2003, 134, 119–25.

Anthony, T; Murray, BW; Sum-Ping, JT; Lenkovsky, F; Vornik, VD; Parker, BJ; et al. Evaluating an evidence-based bundle for preventing surgical site infection. A randomized trial. *Arch Surg.*, 2011, 146, 263–9.

Apisarnthanarak, A; Singh, N; Bandong, AN; et al. Triclosan-coated sutures reduce the risk of surgical site infections: a systematic review and meta-analysis. *Infect Control Hosp Epidemiol*, 2015, 36, 169-179.

Blumetti, J; Luu, M; Sarosi, G; Hartless, K; McFarlin, J; Parker, B; et al. Surgical site infections after colorectal surgery: Do risk factors vary depending on the type of infection considered? *Surgery.*, 2007, 142, 704–11.

Daoud, FC; Edmiston, CE; Jr. Leaper, D. Meta-analysis of prevention of surgical site infections following incision closure with triclosan-coated sutures: robustness to new evidence. *Surg Infect*, 2014, 15, 165-181.

De Jonge, SW; Atema, JJ; Solomkin, JS; et al. Meta-analysis and trial sequential analysis of triclosan-coated sutures for the prevention of surgical-site infection. *Br J Surg*, 2017, 104, 118-133.

Dimick, JB; Chen, SL; Taheri, PA; Henderson, WG; Khuri, SF; Campbell, Jr. DA. Hospital costs associated with surgical complications: A report from the private sector National Surgery Quality Improvement Program. *J Am Coll Surg.*, 2004, 199, 531–7.

Edmiston, CE; Jr. Daoud, FC; Leaper, D. Is there an evidence-based argument for embracing an antimicrobial (triclosan)-coated suture technology to reduce the risk for surgical-site infections? A meta-analysis. *Surgery*, 2013, 154, 89-100.

Guo, J; Pan, L; li, Y; et al. Efficacy of triclosan-coated sutures for reducing risk of surgical site infection in adults: a meta-analysis of randomized clinical trials. *J Surg Res*, 2016, 201, 105-117.

Horan, TC; Andrus, M; Dudeck, MA. CDC/NHSN surveillance definition of health care-associated infection and criteria for specific types of infections in the acute care setting. *Am J Infect Control.*, 2008, 36, 309–32.

Hedrick, TL; Heckman, JA; Smith, RL; Sawyer, RG; Friel, CM; Foley, EF. Efficacy of protocol implementation on incidence of wound infection in colorectal operations. *J Am Coll Surg.*, 2007, 205, 432–8.

Itani, KM; Wilson, SE; Awad, SS; Jensen, EH; Finn, TS; Abramson, MA. Ertapenem versus cefotetan prophylaxis in elective colorectal surgery. *N Engl J Med.*, 2006, 355, 2640–51.

Konstantelias, AA; Andriakopoulou, CS; Mourgela, S. Triclosan-coated sutures for the prevention of surgical-site infections: a meta-analysis. *Acta Chir Belg*, 2017, 117, 137-148.

Leaper, D; Edmiston, CE; Jr. Holy, CE. Meta-analysis of the potential economic impact following introduction of absorbable antimicrobial sutures. *Br J Surg*, 2017, 104, 134-144.

Masini, BD; Stinner, DJ; Waterman, SM; et al. Bacterial adherence to suture materials. *J Surg Educ*, 2011, 68, 101-104.

McMurry, LM; Oethinger, M; Levy, SB. Triclosan targets lipid synthesis. *Nature*, 1998, 394, 531-532.

Murray, BW; Huerta, S; Dineen, S; Anthony, T. Surgical site infection in colorectal surgery: A review of nonpharmacologic tools of prevention. *J AM Coll Surg.*, 2010, 211, 812–22.

Nve Obiang, E; Badia Perez, JM. Surgical site infection: Definition, classification and risk factors. In: Guirao Garriga X, Arias Diaz J. Clinical guidelines of the Spanish Surgical Society. *Surgical infections. Madrid: Aran*, 2006, p. 99–120.

Pastor, C; Artinyan, A; Varma, MG; Kim, E; Gibbs, L; Garcia- Aguilar, J. An increase in compliance with the surgical care improvement project measures does not prevent surgical site infection in colorectal surgery. *Dis Colon Rectum.*, 2010, 53, 24–30.

Ruiz-Tovar, J; Alonso, N; Morales, V; et al. Association between Triclosan-Coated Sutures for Abdominal Wall Closure and Incisional Surgical Site Infection after Open Surgery in Patients Presenting with Fecal Peritonitis: A Randomized Clinical Trial. *Surg Infect*, 2015, 16, 588-594.

Sajid, MS; Craciunas, L; Sains, P; et al. Use of antibacterial sutures for skin closure in controlling surgical site infections: a systematic review of published randomized, controlled trials. *Gastroenterol Rep*, 2013, 1, 42-50.

Serra-Aracil, X; García-Domingo, MI; Parés, D; Espin-Basany, E; Biondo, S; Guirao, X; Orrego, CA; et al. Surgical site infection in elective operations for colorectal cancer after the application of preventive measures. *Arch Surg.*, 2011, 146, 606–12.

Tang, R; Chen, HH; Wang, YL; Changchien, CR; Chen, JS; Hsu, KC; et al. Risk factors for surgical site infection after elective resection of the colon and rectum: A single-center prospective study of 2809 consecutive patients. *Ann Surg.*, 2001, 234, 181–9.

Wang, ZX; Jiang, CP; Cao, Y; et al. Systematic review and meta-analysis of triclosan-coated sutures for the prevention of surgical-site infection. *Br J Surg*, 2013, 100, 465-473.

Wu, X; Kubilay, NZ; Ren, J; et al. Antimicrobial-coated sutures to decrease surgical site infections: a systematic review and meta-analysis. *Eur J Clin Microbiol Infect Dis*, 2017, 36, 19-32.

In: Prophylaxis of Surgical Site Infection … ISBN: 978-1-53615-615-7
Editors: Jaime Ruiz-Tovar et al. © 2019 Nova Science Publishers, Inc.

Chapter 13

WOUND COVER: TOPICAL ANTIBIOTICS OR ANTISEPTICS

Helen Almeida Ponce,[*]MD,
and Pablo Royo Dachary, MD, PhD
Department of Surgery, University of Zaragoza, Zaragoza, Spain

ABSTRACT

Wound coverage is thought to play a role on the prevention of surgical site infection (SSI). Dressings and antiseptics after surgical procedures are widely used and topical antibiotics have been studied by many authors although not included in clinical guidelines. Furthermore, combinations of these three elements are broadly available in clinical practice as an attempt to improve SSI prevention or to potentiate dressings actions on chronic or infected wounds.

Keywords: dressings, topical antibiotics, antiseptics, wounds

---

[*] Corresponding Author's Email: helen.almeida.p@outlook.es.

INTRODUCTION

In general surgery, the acceptable rate of infection following clean surgery is less than 5%, nevertheless, even within cohorts with a low overall risk of infection, some procedures may be at higher risk, and infection rates may be greater than 5% in these high-risk groups.

Wound coverage is a typical conduct throughout the world and common to all surgical and medical disciplines that involve a wound. It could be meant to protect the wound from external aggressive or contaminant agents, to add compression and avoid further bleeding, to manage exudates, to enhance the healing process or to avoid patient's traumatic reaction to the sight of their injuries. The role of wound coverage in the prevention of the surgical site infection (SSI) appears to be obvious, as it implies a physical barrier to external elements, but SSI rates remain the same, indicating that external sources are not the only element behind them and leaving an open door to other preventive actions.

Many initiatives have been suggested and tested in order to prevent or reduce surgical site infection in patients operated on for non-septic processes. In this context, antibiotic infusion is one of multiple measures used to achieve this goal, and its intravenous administration is clearly demonstrated and globalized, same as standard aseptic and antiseptic solutions to reduce the microbial contaminant exposure prior to the surgical procedure. On the other hand, wound coverage following surgical procedures, with elements such as topical antibiotics, antiseptics and dressings is still controversial, and actual guidelines do not include their systematic use after general surgery.

In this chapter we review the existing evidence on the role of wound cover in the prevention of surgical site infection.

WOUND DRESSINGS

Several attributes of an ideal wound dressing have been described according to the British National Formulary, these include: the ability of the dressing to absorb and contain exudate without leakage or strike-through, lack of particulate contaminants left in the wound by the dressing, thermal insulation, impermeability to water and bacteria, suitability of the dressing for use with different skin closure methods, avoidance of wound trauma on dressing removal, frequency with which the dressing needs to be changed, provision of pain relief, cosmesis and comfort, effect on formation of scar tissue, and transparency to aid visualisation of the wound.

Table 1. Simplified classification of wound dressings

Wound dressing	Potential Benefits	Potential risks	Use	Considerations
Wound exposure	Allow follow-up without manipulation	Exposition to environmental contamination	Clean wounds	Some patients may not feel comfortable
Basic dressing				
Absorbent	Simple and inexpensive. Easy to change	Risk of maceration in high exudative wounds	Common wounds	Early (<48h) versus delayed (>48h) change has demonstrated no benefit
Low-adherence	Avoid adhesion to wound tissues	Low absorption capacity	Exposed tissues with risk of adhesion.	They are either non-medicated (e.g., paraffin gauze dressing), or medicated (antibiotics, antiseptics. etc).
Advanced dressings				
Transparent film dressings	Provide a moist healing ambient	Dressing changes are less frequent	Clean wounds	Won't adhere to a moist surface

Table 1. (Continued)

Wound dressing	Potential Benefits	Potential risks	Use	Considerations
Foams	Crates a humid ambient to improve wound healing. Avoid adherence to wound	Dressing changes are less frequent	Moderate exudative wounds	Not recommended in wounds with dead spaces. Certain antiseptics may damage the foam product
Hydrocolloids	Exudate management	Dressing changes are less frequent (every 3-7 days)	High exudative wounds	May cause peri wound maceration
Vacuum assisted	Accelerate wound healing improving vascularization	More expensive	Complex wounds with lack of tissue	Pay attention to bowel exposure
Antimicrobial	Active SSI prophylaxis. Skin decontamination		Potentially infected wounds	Could include antibiotics (e.g., neomycin) or antiseptics (e.g., silver)
Skin adhesives	Act as a barrier	There is no scientific evidence of their benefits	Closure of minor skin wounds and for additional suture support	Contain enbucrilate or octyl 2-cyanoacrylate

Table 1 resumes the wide variety of dressings existing nowadays, as a result of their evolution towards achieving the attributes of an ideal dressing for different types of wounds, potentially improving their capacity to prevent infections, favour the healing process or bettering patients experience.

Basic Dressings

The most frequently used dressing for clean surgical wounds. Basic dressings perfectly fulfil the mission of isolation from external elements. They are simple and inexpensive and allow daily replacements easily. They have an absorbent surface to manage small exudates.

Drawbacks are: 1. their inability to handle highly exudative wounds, which can cause maceration and hinder wound closure; and, 2. allergic reactions or blisters on the skin due to high adherence.

Low adherence basic dressings may contain agents to prevent tissue adhesion, such as vaseline. This is very useful in wounds with exposed tissues, but also greatly diminishes the ability to absorb exudates.

There is no evidence of benefits of early (once every less than 48 hours) versus delayed (once every 48 hours or more) change of basic dressings in terms of wound infection.

Advanced Dressings

They emerge as a result of the extensive research on the different characteristics and requirements of wounds, not only those produced by surgical procedures (clean, contaminated or urgent) but also chronic wounds in diabetic, malnourished, immobilized patients, etc.

The groups most commonly found on general practice and their main characteristics are described in the following section.

Transparent film dressings
They provide a moist healing environment, protect the wound from mechanical trauma and bacterial invasion, act as a blister roof or "second skin" and they are waterproof. Because of their flexibility, they can be used in awkward locations such as joints or skin folds. Transparency makes it easy to visualize the wound bed. Although these dressings can't absorb fluid, they're permeable to moisture allowing one-way passage of carbon dioxide and excess moisture vapor away from the wound. They reduce manipulation as it is not necessary to replace the dressing while the wound shows no signs of infection. Some patients may not feel comfortable with wound visibility. They need healthy skin around the wound because its adhesive properties are deactivated by moisture.

Indications	Contraindications
Partial-thickness wounds with no or minimal drainage When protection is needed for intact skin, for example, protection of bony prominences such as elbows and heels from friction To promote debridement of eschar To protect and secure I.V. catheters To secure another dressing.	Contraindicated in patients with moderate to heavy exudate, third-degree burns, suspected or active infection, fungal infection, or active herpetic lesions. These dressings can cause peri wound maceration. Not recommended for patients with fragile or thin skin, especially elderly patients, or patients receiving steroids, to avoid epidermal stripping or skin tears.

Foams

A porous structure that can absorb fluids into air-filled spaces by capillary action. The most commonly used foam is polyurethane. Silicone foam is less frequently used as the primary absorbent in wound dressing, but it is often applied as an adhesive wound contact layer. These dressings may have variable thickness and can be adhesive or non-adhesive. They are commonly supplied with a film-backing, which has the purpose of providing a water and microbial resistant barrier to the environment. They can be used as primary dressing or secondary dressing in combination with amorphous gels applied to the wound bed to provide moisture. The hydrogels are not absorbed into the foam due to their high viscosity.

Indications	Contraindications
Acute and chronic wounds of both partial and full thickness Medium to heavy exudate.	Certain antiseptics may damage the foam product (e.g., iodine, chlorhexidine, hypochlorite, ether, hydrogen peroxide, oxygenated water, and sodium hypochlorite)

Hydrocolloids:

They contain gel-forming agents (a gelatine or sodium carboxymethylcellulose) held within an adhesive compound, which is laminated in place on a foam or film, generally made of polyurethane. The end product is an advanced wound dressing that resembles an absorbent, flexible wafer, typically both waterproof and self-adhering. Hydrocolloid dressings are occlusive, providing a moist healing environment, autolytic debridement and insulation. Changes should be done every 3 to 7 days depending on wound conditions and type of hydrocolloid.

Indications	Contraindications
Non-infected wounds with scant to moderate drainage Necrotic or granular wound Dry wound Partial- or full-thickness wound Protection of intact skin or a newly healed wound.	Not recommended for wounds with heavy exudate, sinus tracts, or when infection is present Assessment can be difficult if the hydrocolloid dressing is opaque May become dislodged if the wound produces heavy exudate May curl or roll at the edges Upon removal, dressing residue may adhere to the wound bed and there may be an odour May cause peri wound maceration May cause trauma/injury to fragile skin upon removal May cause hypergranulation

Impregnated dressings
Gauze, bandage, etc. treated with a special chemical agent that promotes increased wound healing and a generally more sterile environment. These compounds must be paired with a secondary dressing, as they are generally non-adherent to most wound beds. There are several preferred impregnating mixtures, and each one has its own use and benefits. 1. Silver impregnated dressings: silver is utilized to help reduce the spread of bacteria and other harmful contaminants. Most often, physicians will pair silver with alginate or foam dressings, which improve its bacteria-fighting capabilities. They can be used on almost any wound, including heel abrasions and various ulcers. 2. Honey impregnated dressings: Like silver, honey has broad-spectrum applications. The acid found in honey causes an uptick in oxygenation, which makes the wound bed all but inhospitable for most forms of bacteria. It's worth noting, though, that there are several different kinds of honey – like fireweed, sage and orange blossom – and each variety is uniquely potent as an antimicrobial agent. 3. Iodine impregnated dressings: This chemical is used extensively as a powerful disinfectant. Among a number of trials, iodine worked best in healing chronic ulcers and low-level burns, as the chemical was adept at destroying bacteria in these unique wound beds. 4. Methylene blue dressings: methyl blue is proven against several bacteria, including vancomycin-resistant enterococcus. This wound agent is normally paired with gentian violet which is best at combating a variety of fungal strains. Hydrofera Blue is one of the most popular dressings featuring this methyl-gentian combination. This dressing is used to treat everything, from **diabetic ulcers,** to wounds that come as a result of acute respiratory distress syndrome. Hydrofera Blue is noted for being more absorbent than other dressings, especially silver and foam, and doesn't hinder growth factor activity. 5. Antibiotic dressings: they are non-toxic and can work effectively on the target sites without damaging hosts tissues. Some of the most commonly used are quinolones such as ciprofloxacin, ofloxacin, levofloxacin, etc; gentamycin, doxycycline, nitrofurantoin, etc.
Vacuum-assisted closure (VAC):
This device decreases air pressure on the wound. This can help the wound heal faster by gently removing fluid from the wound over time, reducing swelling, favouring wound´s cleansing and removing bacteria. A wound VAC also helps pull the edges of the wound together. And it may stimulate the growth of new tissue that helps the wound close. A wound vacuum system has several parts. A foam or gauze dressing is put directly on the wound. An adhesive film covers and seals the dressing and wound. A drainage tube leads from under the adhesive film and connects to a portable vacuum pump. This pump removes air pressure over the wound either constantly, or in cycles. The dressing is changed every 24 to 72 hours.

Indications	Contraindications and risks
Highly exudative wounds that require frequent changes of other types of dressings. Wounds healing by first or second intention provided that they have no bleeding or exposed bowels	Negative pressure should not be used in wounds with active or known risk of: Bleeding Enteric fistula

Skin adhesives
Cyanoacrylate tissue adhesives combine cyanoacetate and formaldehyde in a heat vacuum along with a base to form a liquid monomer. When the monomer comes in contact with moisture on the skin's surface, it chemically changes into a polymer that binds to the top epithelial layer. This polymer forms a cyanoacrylate bridge, binding the two wound edges together and allowing normal healing to

occur below. The conversion from monomer to polymer occurs rapidly, preventing seepage of the adhesive below the wound margins, as long as the edges are well apposed. Heat is often generated during the change from monomer to polymer, and this heat may be felt on occasion by patients during application to the skin. Cyanoacrylates have also been shown to have antimicrobial properties. The adhesive acts as its own water-resistant bandage, and no added coverings are needed. Patients may shower normally and pat the area dry. The adhesive will spontaneously peel off in five to 10 days.

Indications	Contraindications
Wounds healing on first intention Non-exudative wounds with clean edges	High risk of wound exudate or wound infection Topical antibiotics should not be applied to the closed wound for this would break down the adhesive and cause early peeling.

Studies to assess the effectiveness of dressings in the prevention of SSI have compared wound exposure to basic and advanced dressings, and basic contact dressings to advanced, antimicrobial and adhesive dressings. No recommendation based on evidence has emerged from the existing data.

Wound Cover versus Wound Exposure

It is uncertain whether there is a difference in SSI risk between basic wound dressing and wound exposure. Two trials were carried (Law in 1987 and Phan in 1993), comparing both clean and potentially contaminated surgery, with a combined total of 409 patients. No differences were found in SSI in the comparison groups. Both trials have a very low certainty evidence and a high risk of bias and their findings are summarized in Table 2.

Table 2. Wound exposure vs basic wound dressing

Author, year	Type of surgery	No.	SSI in covered vs exposed wounds	RR
Law, 1987	Clean	112	3/59 (5%) vs 1/53 (2%)	0.37 95% CI 0,4-3,46
Phan, 1993	Potentially contaminated	297	21/102 (21%) vs 29/105 (28%)	1.34 95% CI 0,82 – 2,19

In 2011, Siah et al. compared a silver dressing with wound exposure in 166 participants undergoing various types of elective colorectal surgery classified as clean/contaminated. No significant differences were found, as 8/83 (10%) in the exposed wound group developed SSI, compared with 1/83 (1%) in the silver-dressed wound group (RR: 8.00, 95% 1.02 to 62.55) with evidence of very low certainty, downgraded once for risk of bias and twice for imprecision by the Cochrane research team.

Dressings Compared with Other Type of Dressings

Many studies have been conducted comparing multiple kinds of dressings, in order to determine effectiveness in the prevention of SSI, and other characteristics such as ease of removal, effect on pain, costs, etc., but, as with other broad fields, heterogenicity in measurement scales and reported results, makes it difficult to draw conclusions.

Basic Wound Contact Dressings versus Film Dressings

Eight trials including 1089 patients (pooling all trials), compared a basic wound contact dressing with a film dressing. Five of these trials evaluated wounds resulting from 'clean' surgical procedures (Cosker 2005; De Win 1998; Law 1987; Moshakis 1984; Wynne 2004). According to the Cochrane revision on the subject, for clean surgery *"There is uncertain evidence on the risk of SSI between basic wound contact-dressed wounds and film-dressed wounds (RR 1.34; 95% CI 0.70 to 2.55); very low certainty evidence downgraded once for risk of bias and twice for imprecision."*

Two studies evaluated wounds resulting from surgical procedures with mixed, or unclear, contamination classifications. The trials included a variety of basic wound contact dressings including gauze and surgical absorbents. Similarly, whilst the comparators were all film dressings of different brands. Table 3 summarizes de results of these two trials.

Table 3. Basic wound contact dressing *versus* film dressing

Author, year	Type of surgery	No.	SSI in contact vs film dressings	RR
Gardezi, 1983	Clean/contaminated	100	6/50 (12%) vs 3/50 (6%)	0.50 95% CI 0.13- 1.89
Rohde, 1979	Unclear	90	24/46 (52%) vs 14/44 (32%)	0.61; 95% CI 0.36 to 1.02. In favour of the film dressing.

Basic Contact Wound Dressings Compared with Hydrocolloid Dressings

Six trials with a pooled total of 792 participants investigated the effect of a basic wound contact dressing compared with a hydrocolloid dressing (Holm 1998; Michie 1994; Persson 1995; Shinohara 2008; Wikblad 1995; Wynne 2004). The basic wound contact dressings were predominantly gauze.

Michie, Wikblad y Wynne described results on SSI after clean surgery, but each author on different terms, hence, no pooled data analysis was possible and there is no joint conclusion available; Wynne found no differences between hydrocolloid-dressed 6/267; (2%) and basic wound contact-dressed wounds 6/243; (3%) (RR 0.91; 95% CI 0.30 to 2.78).

The pooled data from the three trials that presented SSI data on contaminated surgery (Holm 1998; Persson 1995; Shinohara 2008) showed no differences between groups with a RR 0.57; 95% CI 0.22 to 1.51.

Basic Wound Contact Dressings Compared with Silver Dressings

Eight trials with a pooled total of 1959 patients, examined differences between these two types of dressings. Two authors included participants undergoing clean surgery (Dickinson Jennings 2015; Politano 2011). Six studies compared the use of a basic wound dressing with a silver-containing dressing in surgery at risk of contamination. Four studies involved colorectal surgery (Biffi 2012; Kriegar 2011; Prather 2011; Ruiz-Tovar 2015). Bennett randomized 524 participants who had undergone a caesarean section and Ozaki randomized 500 people undergoing a non-emergency surgical procedure for peripheral vascular disease.

After analysing data of the two groups (clean surgery = 2 studies and potentially contaminated surgery = 6 studies) the Cochrane revision on the subject concludes that it is uncertain whether silver dressings increase or reduce SSI for either group with a RR 1.11; 0.47 to 2.62 for clean surgery and RR 0.83; 95% CI 0.51 to 1.37 for the potentially contaminated group.

Basic Wound Contact Dressing Compared with Non-Silver Antimicrobial Dressings

Martin-Trapero randomized 197 participants undergoing elective laparoscopic cholecystectomy to a basic wound contact or a Phenilmetil biguanide (PHMB) impregnated antimicrobial dressing. SSI in the wound contact dressing group was 5% (5/101); while the PHMB dressing-treated group had 1% (1/96). As the 95% CIs are wide and include benefits (in terms of reduced SSI risk) and harms (in terms of increased SSI risks) differences between the two groups remain unclear (RR 0.21, 95% CI 0.03 to 1.77).

Conclusion

Authors of the Cochrane revision conclude that there is insufficient evidence to determine whether covering surgical wounds healing by primary intention, with wound dressings, reduces the risk of surgical site infections (SSIs), or if any particular type of wound dressing reduces the risk of infections more than another. The review also failed to demonstrate any clear advantage of one dressing type over another (or wound exposure) for improved scarring, pain control, patient acceptability or ease of removal.

TOPICAL ANTIBIOTICS

The role of topical antibiotics has not been consistently supported by evidence and, therefore, they are not included in current guidelines for the prevention of SSI. There are thought to be benefits in using antibiotics topically rather than orally, or intravenously, as topical antibiotics act only on the area of the body where they are applied, there is less likelihood of unwanted effects that affect the whole body, such as nausea and diarrhea. Topical antibiotics are also thought to reduce the chances of bacterial resistance.

The most common method of application of topical antibiotics is in the form of an ointment. Other possible delivery methods include cream, lotion, solution, gel, tincture, foam, paste, powder, and impregnated dressings. An ointment base classically contains 80% oil and 20% water, and therefore is more occlusive and will drive the medication into the skin more rapidly than a solution or cream base; thus, ointments are an optimal delivery method for topical antibiotics.

In 2016 the Cochrane Database of Systematic Reviews selected 10 randomized controlled trials, including 6466 patients, assessing the effectiveness of topical antibiotics on preventing SSI, to determine whether the application of topical antibiotics to surgical wounds that are healing by primary intention reduces the incidence of SSI and the incidence of adverse outcomes (allergic contact dermatitis, infections with patterns of antibiotic resistance and anaphylaxis). All forms of topical antibiotics were included (creams, impregnated dressings, ointments, etc) provided that their application followed wound closure by primary intention. Silver and antiseptic impregnated dressings were excluded given that these substances did not match the definition of antibiotic.

The results of this systematic review are summarized in the following sections as they gather the most recent evidence on the subject.

Topical Antibiotic versus No Topical Antibiotic

The results of eight trials were pooled (5427 participants) using a random-effects model. The -no topical antibiotic- group included: inert ointment (Dire 1995; Dixon 2006; Heal 2009; Smack 1996) and no treatment (Caro 1967; Dixon 2006; Gilmore 1973a; Kamath 2005;

Khalighi 2014). There were *fewer SSIs with topical antibiotics than without* (RR 0.61; 95% CI 0.42 to 0.87). There was an absolute risk difference of 20 fewer SSIs per 1000 patients (95% CI 7 fewer to 31 fewer) and a *number needed to treat to benefit* (NNTB) with topical antibiotics to avoid one additional SSI (NNT) of 50. There was moderate inter study heterogeneity (I^2 = 44%). The quality of evidence for this outcome was graded as moderate, downgraded once for the proportion of the information from studies at high risk of selection bias, as this was sufficient to affect the interpretation of the results, a sensitivity analysis was performed to examine the effect of removing the studies at high risk of bias on I^2 and RR (Caro 1967; Dixon 2006; Gilmore 1973). The effect estimate was robust to removal of high risk of bias studies (RR 0.49, 95% CI 0.35 to 0.67; 3026 participants; 5 studies; I2 = 0%).

No clear difference between groups for risk of allergic contact dermatitis was found (RR 3.94, 95% CI 0.46 to 34.00).

Topical Antibiotic versus Topical Antibiotic

One study (99 participants) was a head-to-head comparison of mupirocin and neomycin (Hood 2004). There was no clear evidence of a difference between mupirocin and neomycin in risk of SSI (RR 0.20; 95% CI 0.01 to 4.14; P = 0.3). The quality of evidence for this outcome was rated as very low. Another study was a four-arm trial; two arms of which were antibiotic arms combination ointment (neomycin sulphate, bacitracin zinc, and polymyxin B sulphate) versus bacitracin zinc (Dire 1995). Comparison of the results for these two arms showed no clear evidence of a difference in risk of SSI (RR 0.83; 95% CI 0.26 to 2.63; 219 participants, P = 0.75).

These two trials did not compare similar topical antibiotics and so were not pooled. The quality of evidence of this outcome was rated as very low and was downgraded twice for risk of bias and once for imprecision.

There was no information available for the outcomes of allergic contact dermatitis or anaphylaxis for either study.

Topical Antibiotics versus Antiseptic

Five trials that compared topical antibiotics with antiseptics were pooled (1299 participants) to examine effects on risk of SSI. There were fewer SSIs in those treated with topical antibiotics than with antiseptics (RR 0.49, 95% CI 0.30 to 0.80). This difference reflected an absolute difference in risk of 43 fewer cases of SSI per 1000 people treated with topical antibiotics instead of antiseptics (95% CI 17 fewer to 59 fewer per 1000; NNTB of 24). There was minor inter study heterogeneity ($I^2 = 12\%$). The quality of evidence for this outcome was rated as moderate and was downgraded. A sensitivity analysis was performed to examine the effect of removing the studies at high risk of bias on I^2 and RR (Gilmore 1973a; Iselin 1990). The overall effect was robust to removal of the high risk of bias studies (RR 0.39, 95% CI 0.20 to 0.76) and heterogeneity was reduced ($I^2 = 0\%$).

Two trials (541 participants) compared the effects of topical antibiotics and antiseptics on the rates of allergic contact dermatitis. Pooled analysis indicated no clear evidence of a difference (RR 0.97, 95% CI 0.52 to 1.82; I2 = 0%, P = 0.92). One of the two studies was at high risk of bias and the other was at unclear risk of bias. The overall quality of the evidence was rated as very low

CONCLUSION

Topical antibiotics probably prevent surgical site infection (SSI) whether compared with antiseptic or to no topical antibiotic (moderate quality evidence). The Cochrane review only identified studies involving clean (class1), clean contaminated (class 2), and contaminated (class 3) surgery, and no conclusions regarding dirty-contaminated (class 4) surgery can be drawn.

In clean surgery, where the baseline infection rate is already low, and the absolute risk reduction in SSI is smaller, the use of topical antibiotics is probably not justified. In classes 2 and 3, the actual reduction in the rate of infection was 4.3% on average when the use of topical antibiotic was compared with antiseptic, and 2% when compared to no treatment, this means it would require 24 patients, on average, to be treated with topical antibiotics instead of antiseptics, and 50 patients to be treated with topical antibiotics, compared to no treatment, in order to prevent one wound infection.

The Cochrane Database review was unable to draw conclusions regarding the effects of topical antibiotics on adverse outcomes, such as allergic contact dermatitis, due to lack of statistical power. It was also unable to draw conclusions regarding the impact of increasing topical antibiotic use on antibiotic resistance.

ANTISEPTICS

The application of antiseptics such as povidone or chlorhexidine at the end of a surgical procedure, after wound closure and prior to the application of any kind of dressing, is widely extended, though it is very hard to find any scientific base to this practice. Regardless of the background of this conduct, after tissue manipulation, bleeding, etc it seems only logical to repeat antiseptic procedures if not to reduce SSI, at least to improve wounds appearance.

Antiseptics are chemical agents that reduce the microbial population on the skin. They should gather certain attributes to be consider ideal, such as: kill all bacteria, fungi, viruses, protozoa, tubercle bacilli and spores; be non-toxic; be hypoallergenic; be safe to use in all body regions; not to be absorbed; have residual activity; be safe for repetitive use.

Several antiseptic agents are available for preoperative preparation of skin at the incision site. Most commonly used include iodine as iodine, povidone iodine, cadexomer iodine or povidone; chlorhexidine as polyhexamethylene biguanide or chlorhexidine. Some authors also include silver as an antiseptic or antimicrobial since it does not meet the criteria that defines antibiotics, but it is not used for skin preparation.

Studies that asses the effectivity of antiseptics versus topical antibiotics or dressings impregnated with these substances compared with other types of dressings are detailed in the sections above.

REFERENCES

Atiyeh, Bishara S., Saad A. Dibo, y Shady N. Hayek. 2009. "Wound Cleansing, Topical Antiseptics and Wound Healing." *International Wound Journal* 6 (6): 420-30. https://doi.org/10.1111/j.1742-481X.2009.00639.x.

Berger, R. S., A. S. Pappert, P. S. Van Zile, y W. E. Cetnarowski. 2000. "A Newly Formulated Topical Triple-Antibiotic Ointment Minimizes Scarring." *Cutis* 65 (6): 401-4.

Dumville, Jo C, Trish A Gray, Catherine J Walter, Catherine A Sharp, Tamara Page, Rhiannon Macefield, Natalie Blencowe, Thomas KG Milne, Barnaby C Reeves, y Jane Blazeby. 2016. "Dressings for the Prevention of Surgical Site Infection." Cochrane Wounds Group. *Cochrane Database of Systematic Reviews.* https://doi.org/10.1002/14651858.CD003091.pub4.

Dumville, Jo C, Emma McFarlane, Peggy Edwards, Allyson Lipp, Alexandra Holmes, y Zhenmi Liu. 2015. "Preoperative Skin Antiseptics for Preventing Surgical Wound Infections after Clean Surgery." Cochrane Wounds Group. *Cochrane Database of Systematic Reviews.* https://doi.org/10.1002/14651858.CD003949.pub4.

Heal, Clare F, Jennifer L Banks, Phoebe D Lepper, Evangelos Kontopantelis, y Mieke L van Driel. 2016. "Topical Antibiotics for Preventing Surgical Site Infection in Wounds Healing by Primary Intention." Cochrane Wounds Group. *Cochrane Database of Systematic Reviews.* https://doi.org/10.1002/14651858.CD011426.pub2.

Hirsch, Tobias, Hans-Martin Seipp, Frank Jacobsen, Ole Goertz, Hans-Ulrich Steinau, y Lars Steinstraesser. 2010. "Antiseptics in Surgery." *Eplasty* 10 (may): e39.

Kowalczuk, J. 2006. "British National Formulary for Children 2005." *Quality and Safety in Health Care* 15 (1): 76-76. https://doi.org/10.1136/qshc.2005.016881.

Kramer, Axel, Joachim Dissemond, Simon Kim, Christian Willy, Dieter Mayer, Roald Papke, Felix Tuchmann, y Ojan Assadian. 2018. "Consensus on Wound Antisepsis: Update 2018." *Skin Pharmacology and Physiology* 31 (1): 28-58. https://doi.org/10.1159/000481545.

Law, N. W., y H. Ellis. 1987. "Exposure of the Wound--a Safe Economy in the NHS." *Postgraduate Medical Journal* 63 (735): 27-28.

Lee, Ingi, Rajender K. Agarwal, Bruce Y. Lee, Neil O. Fishman, y Craig A. Umscheid. 2010. "Systematic Review and Cost Analysis Comparing Use of Chlorhexidine with Use of Iodine for Preoperative Skin Antisepsis to Prevent Surgical Site Infection." *Infection Control & Hospital Epidemiology* 31 (12): 1219-29. https://doi.org/10.1086/657134.

Phan, M., P. Van der Auwera, G. Andry, M. Aoun, G. Chantrain, R. Deraemaecker, P. Dor, D. Daneau, P. Ewalenko, y F. Meunier. 1993. "Wound Dressing in Major Head and Neck Cancer Surgery: A Prospective Randomized Study of Gauze Dressing vs Sterile Vaseline Ointment." *European Journal of Surgical Oncology: The Journal of the European Society of Surgical Oncology and the British Association of Surgical Oncology* 19 (1): 10-16.

Ruiz Tovar, Jaime, y Josep M. Badia. 2014. "Prevention of surgical site infection in abdominal surgery. A critical review of the evidence." *Cirugía Española* 92 (4): 223-31. https://doi.org/10.1016/j.ciresp.2013.08.003.

Ruiz-Tovar, Jaime, Carolina Llavero, Vicente Morales, y Carlos Gamallo. 2015. "Total Occlusive Ionic Silver-Containing Dressing vs Mupirocin Ointment Application vs Conventional Dressing in Elective Colorectal Surgery: Effect on Incisional Surgical Site Infection." *Journal of the American College of Surgeons* 221 (2): 424-29. https://doi.org/10.1016/j.jamcollsurg.2015.04.019.

Toon, Clare D, Charnelle Lusuku, Rajarajan Ramamoorthy, Brian R Davidson, y Kurinchi Selvan Gurusamy. 2015. "Early versus Delayed Dressing Removal after Primary Closure of Clean and Clean-Contaminated Surgical Wounds." Cochrane Wounds Group. *Cochrane Database of Systematic Reviews*. https://doi.org/10.1002/14651858.CD010259.pub3.

Chapter 14

BUNDLES

Camilo J. Castellón Pavón[1], MD, PhD,
Sonia Morales Artero[2], MD, Elena Larraz Mora[2], MD,
Jaime Ruiz-Tovar[3], MD, PhD
and Manuel Durán Poveda[1], MD, PhD

[1]Department of General Surgery, Hospital "Rey Juan Carlos,"
Mostoles, Madrid, Spain
King Juan Carlos University
[2]Department of General Surgery, Hospital "El Escorial,"
Madrid, Spain
Francisco de Vitoria University
[3]Department of General Surgery, Hospital "Rey Juan Carlos,"
Mostoles, Madrid, Spain
Alfonso X University, Madrid, Spain

ABSTRACT

Care bundles are a collection of evidence-based clinical practices which include a reduced number of interventions that have shown to improve patient outcome for a particular symptom, procedure or treatment. Used together as a cluster, the result is superior to the addition of individual outcomes.

The concept of care bundle was first developed in the US by the Institute for Healthcare Improvement (IHI) in 2001 to improve clinical effectiveness in patients treated in intensive care units. Since then, many other care bundles have been implemented and used for a variety of indications.

Surgical site infection (SSI) is the most common and preventable hospital-acquired infection and is associated with higher hospital stay, mortality, hospital readmissions and health costs. Bundles have successfully reduced SSI after surgical procedures, especially in colorectal surgery. High bundle compliance correlates with better results in terms of SSI rates. There are many interventions reported in different implemented bundles, some of them with lower clinical evidence. Future studies of bundles will help to assess the best strategies and describe compliance methodology to improve quality of care in surgical patients.

Keywords: surgical site infection, prophylaxis, bundles

INTRODUCTION

During the last decades, several agencies and international institutions have implemented different measures and programs in order to improve patient security and quality of care. A care bundle is a set of standard clinical practices used to reduce potential complications and to improve the evolution of patients with a certain symptom or receiving certain treatment with high inherent risks [1]. Results are better when this set of measures are implemented altogether, than the sum of each measure used individually. Not every clinical situation requires the use of a care bundle, so each centre must establish their indications according to a type of intervention, describe the critical points which grant their implementation and choose the bundles which better adjust to their resources. Bundles are complementary to enhanced recovery pathways (ERP) but have important differences with a checklist [2]. A checklist is very helpful for ensuring safe and reliable care. The elements in a checklist are often a combination of useful and important tasks or actions, but not evidence-based changes. A checklist may also have many elements. Some elements are not essential, so there may be no effect on the patient when they are not completed. On the other hand, each element in a bundle is relatively independent and the changes are all necessary and all sufficient [2, 3]. When an element is missed, the patient is at much greater risk for serious complications. The changes are based on randomized controlled trials (level 1 of evidence). There should be no controversy involved, no debate or discussion about bundle elements. Each step is a simple and straightforward process that should be successfully completed. The changes involve "all or nothing" measurement [2]. Also, bundle changes occur in the same time and space continuum: at a specific time and in a specific place.

The term care bundle was first introduced in 2001 by the Institute for Healthcare Improvement (IHI) with the aim of reducing individual variability in clinical practice and improving the management of the healthcare process in critical patients [2, 3]. In 2002, Berenholtz et al. identified six evidence-based interventions which were able to reduce morbimortality of patients in intensive care units: effective assessment of pain, appropriate use of blood transfusions, prevention of ventilator-associated pneumonia (VAP), appropriate sedation, peptic ulcer prophylaxis and deep vein thrombosis prophylaxis [4]. The IHI ventilator bundle and the IHI central line bundle were the first bundles developed and were included in IHI´s 100.00 lives campaign and 5 million lives campaign [3, 5]. More than 4000 US hospitals were enrolled in the campaigns between 2004 and 2008. As a result, 65 hospitals reported spending one year or more without a case of VAP and 35 hospitals reported six months or more without a central line-associated bloodstream infection in an ICU. In August 2002, the Centres for Medicare and Medicaid Services (CMS) and the Centres for Disease Control and Prevention (CDC) implemented the National Surgical Infection Prevention (SIP) Project [6-7]. Later, in 2006, the Surgical Care Improvement Project (SCIP) was developed, as an evolution of the SIP [8]. SCIP includes measures that can be implemented to reduce surgical infectious and non-infectious complications in more prevalent major interventions. Since then, the concept care bundle has developed and expanded, recording several prophylactic evidence-based clinical measures intended to prevent complications in high risk situations, such as the critical patient, obstetrics, orthopaedic surgery [9] and abdominal surgery. Every implemented measure must be based on strict scientific knowledge, follow a protocol and results must be evaluable, in order to improve the healthcare process. Many bundles have been published, sometimes with contradictory results because of the great variability in the elements used for each bundle and their different application in each centre [10]. Institutions that desire to improve their healthcare quality need to implement a bigger amount of care bundles, in order to determine which are the most effective and appropriate evidence-based measures to apply on each specific clinical situation. Bundles should be expected to evolve over time because of new evidence, focusing on the aim of improvement [11].

IMPLEMENTATION OF CARE BUNDLES

A bundle is a specific tool with clear parameters. The following steps have been recommended for the development of a care bundle [1, 11]:

1. Identify the subject.
2. Identify a bundle of three to five evidence-based interventions with strong clinician agreement. Bundle elements should be descriptive rather than prescriptive. Bundles with too many elements are unworkable and ineffective.
3. Identify the relevant research supporting the practices.
4. Categorize the research by quality.
5. Delete practices for which there is inadequate evidence.
6. Measure compliance as "all or none." Compliance with the bundle means completion of every element, with no score given for partial completion.
7. Measure related outcomes to ascertain the effects of the changes in the delivery system.

A critical aspect for effective implementation is to verify adequate bundle compliance and to add it to the quality culture of medical departments. Changing culture is an arduous process, but it is mandatory as part of the bundle to ensure success. A multidisciplinary care team develops the bundle. Successful implementation requires engagement from all the staff involved. Each member of the team must know the importance of every action, must apply all the interventions on every patient and must assume proactive participation, looking for potential improvement. Implementation has to be dynamic and clinical results continuously examined, based on Deming´s PDCA cycle (Plan-Do-Check-Act). Standardization of the care process into a bundle should be expected to reach a very high level of reliability. A realistic first step is to aim for 80 or 90% success rate, then identify and mitigate defects in order to achieve more than 95% reliability [3, 11].

Many different care bundles have been developed in surgical patients, mainly focused on management of sepsis and septic shock and on prevention of hospital-acquired infection [11]: ventilator-associated pneumonia, catheter-related bloodstream infection and prevention of surgical site infection (SSI). In this chapter we are going to focus on preventive surgical site infection bundles (SSIB).

SURGICAL SITE INFECTION BUNDLES

Nosocomial infections are a very important health problem. SSI has become the most common hospital-acquired infection (HAI) in recent years, accounting for almost 40% of infections reported to the Centre for Disease Control (CDC) and 20% of all HAI [12, 14]. The incidence of SSI is 2-5% in patients undergoing surgery in the United States [14, 15]. Nevertheless, incidences reported are variable, depending on the definition of SSI, type of intervention, wound type and surveillance compliance [16].

There are different definitions of SSI, based on International Classification of Diseases (ICD) coding (10th revision), CDC criteria, NINSS modification of the CDC definition, and Current Procedural

Terminology and ASEPSIS score [13, 17-19]. Choosing an optimal definition is difficult. A definition that is too sensitive would overestimate the infection rates, while a definition that lacks sensitivity would not identify avoidable infections. The most widely used definition of SSI has been provided by CDC [20]. In 1992, the CDC definition of infection at the surgical site expanded from "wound infection" to "surgical site infection" [17, 19]. Surgical site infections are defined as infections whose onset is within 30 days after a surgical intervention without a prosthetic implant or within 90 days after a prosthetic surgery [20]. SSIs are classified by depth and tissue spaces involved. Superficial incisional SSI only involves the skin or subcutaneous tissue and often does not require hospitalization. Deep incisional SSI involves the fascia and/or muscular layers and organ space SSI involves any part of the body opened or manipulated during a procedure, excluding the previously mentioned layers [13, 19]. Deep incisional and organ space infections are considered "complex" SSIs. In most series, complex SSI represents about one-third to one-half of SSIs, although this varies depending on the procedure. Complex SSIs typically require re-hospitalization, drainage and systemic antimicrobial therapy [13, 19].

Gastrointestinal procedures are the most common cause of SSI due to the presence of intraluminal bacteria. According to the National Healthcare Safety Network, rates of SSI following bile duct, liver or pancreatic surgery are as high as 10% of the procedures, while rates after colorectal surgery are approximately 5% [21].

SSIs are associated with longer hospital stay and higher mortality, hospital readmissions, and requirements for home health care and supplies [12, 14]. These consequences translate to higher health costs [12].

Aetiology of SSI is multifactorial [13, 19]. There are patient risk factors, such as obesity, advanced age, diabetes mellitus, malnutrition, tobacco use, chronic systemic disease, drug and alcohol abuse, steroid use, immunosuppressive therapies, colonization with virulent/resistant organisms, remote infections and long hospital stay before the operation [12]. Procedure-related factors include timing of surgery (emergency *vs* elective), surgical technique (open approach *vs* laparoscopic procedures), wound class, complexity of surgery and length of operation. Other important perioperative factors are antimicrobial prophylaxis, mechanical bowel preparation (MBP) before colorectal surgery, hand hygiene, surgical attire and other barrier devices, skin antisepsis and method of hair removal at the surgical site before the incision, sterilization of equipment, use of laminar airflow in the operating room (OR), adherence to surgical aseptic/sterile technique, contamination with enteric contents, foreign bodies/implants, supplemental oxygen, maintenance of normothermia, minimize ischemia and red cell transfusions, use of antibiotic sutures and glycemic control [8, 10, 12, 22].

SSI is considered the most preventable HAI (50-60%) [14, 23], having the potential to be reduced by a bundle approach, as there are many associated risk factors to target and there are a considerable number of evidence-based interventions. Many institutions have developed strategies to reduce SSI risk including the World Health Organization (WHO), the Surgical Care Improvement Project (SCIP), Joint Commission National Patient Safety Goals, the American College of Surgeons (ACS) and Surgical Infection Society (SIS), the Healthcare Infection Control Practices Advisory Committee (HICPAC), the Society for Healthcare Epidemiology of America (SHEA), the National Institute for Health and Care Experience (NICE), the National Health Service Scotland (NHSS) and the Canadian Patient Safety Institute [13, 14, 24]. The SCIP measures focused on SSI were the use of glucose control in cardiac surgery patients, proper hair removal at the surgical site and maintenance of normothermia [8]. Several studies have demonstrated that adherence to SCIP measures has improved over the implementation period, but only a few assessed whether adherence has resulted in reduced surgical infection rates and there is minimal evidence to support that SCIP adherence improves surgical outcomes [22, 23, 25]. Besides, not all the measures have been equally effective [25]. Experts have recommended that the focus should now be placed on additional strategies that go beyond SCIP recommendations [22, 26, 27]. Nowadays there are five core evidence-based interventions widely accepted by international institutions: appropriate hair removal, antibiotic prophylaxis, chlorhexidine-alcohol-based skin preparation, normothermia and perioperative glycemic control [28, 29]. Many other measures are recommended by some institutions but not by others, and more randomized clinical trial evidence is needed to support them. Specific and more comprehensive bundle approaches to SSI prevention are succeeding in reducing SSI rates in many procedure categories, especially in colorectal [30-41], hepatic and pancreatic surgery [42, 43].

Though in one randomized trial the bundle resulted in an increase in SSI [44], most SSIB in colorectal surgery (CRS) clearly result in a significant reduction of SSI. However, the Hawthorne effect has to be taken into account when analysing the results in most reported studies. It is worth noting that there is no consensus about the most effective measures, and it is difficult to determine the contribution of each element to SSI reduction, because of the complex interaction between patient, disease, procedure, surgeon, institution factors, and simultaneous synergic strategies applied at the same time. Many centres have adopted the evidence-based SCIP measures as core strategies adding other enclosed measures, sometimes incorporating simple interventions considered "good practices" with less supporting evidence but in order to ensure high compliance [28, 29]. As a result, numerous bundles have been reported including multiple elements in the preoperative, intraoperative and postoperative phases (Table 1). Two meta-analyses have confirmed the benefit of bundling multiple interventions to reduce SSI rates after CRS. In a review of 13 trials (8,515 patients), Tanner et al. observed that SSI rate decreased from 15,1% to 7% [45]. None of the studies included identical SSIB and full implementation was limited. Zywot et al. reviewed 23 bundle studies (15,557 patients) and found an overall SSI reduction of 40%, with 44% for superficial SSI and 34% for organ-space SSI [46]. Two thirds of the studies included identified statistically significant decrease in SSI rates, ranging from 27% to 69%. The studies with higher bundle compliance had significantly lower SSI rates and health costs.

Table 1. Elements in different SSI care bundles in colorectal surgery

	Anthony (2011)	Bull (2011)	Cima (2013)	Crolla (2012)	Lutfiyya (2012)	Waits (2014)	Keenan (2015)	Yamamoto (2015)	Ghuman (2015)	Connolly (2015)	Tanner (2016)	DeHaas (2016)	Weisser (2018)	Hoang (2018)	Ruiz-Tovar (2018)	Edmiston (2018)
Appropriate hair removal	X					X	X				X	X	X	X		
Antibiotic prophylaxis		X	X	X	X	X	X		X	X	X	X	X	X	X	
Skin preparation			X	X	X		X			X	X	X	X	X	X	X
Normothermia	X	X		X	X	X	X		X	X	X	X	X	X	X	
Glucose control		X			X	X	X			X	X			X		
Wound protectors	X						X					X				
Antibiotic sutures								X		X		X				
Limited OR "traffic"	X			X			X			X						X
MBP + oral antibiotic	X					X	X		MBP	MBP		X	X	X		X
Sterile closure tray			X				X		X	X		X	X	X		
Gloves changes			X		X		X		X	X		X				
Wound irrigation					X			X	X							
Wound sealants								X								
Topical antibiotic																
Supplemental oxygen	X	X									X			X	X	
Antibacterial dressing											X					
Wound care			X						X			X				
Reduction of intravenous fluids during operation	X														X	
Systemic blood pressure maintenance		X														
MRSA screening											X					X
Checklist fulfillment															X	
Intraperitoneal irrigation with antibiotic solution															X	
Smoking cessation					X											

Bundle implementation at Mayo Clinic was associated with more than 50% reduction in SSIs (from 9,8% to 4%) [30]. Hoang et al. achieved a significant reduction of SSI rates after CRS (9,4% to 4,7%) with a bundle of eleven elements [41]. The Michigan Surgical Collaborative group reported a direct correlation between compliance with bundle implementation and colorectal SSI rate [33]. Compliance was more common in a selected group of "low-risk" patients undergoing elective operations. An Australian study found a 50% reduction of SSI after CRS, but it was no statistically significant [47]. However, the bundle compliance in this study was very low (21%) and the power was insufficient to draw definitive conclusions [34, 47]. Keenan et al. also observed SSI reduction after implementation of a bundle as part of an ERP [35]. Perioperative Quality Initiative (POQI) workgroup in Durham also recommended SSIB implementation as part of a colorectal ERP [48]. Weiser et al. reported great reduction of superficial and deep but not organ-space SSI, with the implementation of a care bundle differing from others in the inclusion of a colorectal SSI prediction tool that informs surgeons about the SSI risk before surgery, what may influence the wound closure method chosen in higher-risk patients [32].

Crolla et al. reported 36% reduction of SSI with a SSIB paying attention on the number of door openings in the OR [34]. Their target was less than ten door movements per hour and the compliance rate was up to 80% at the end of the study. For the authors, the door openings strongly correlate with higher noise levels during the surgical procedure that somehow are associated with SSI due to a lack of concentration, a stressful environment and a changing behaviour of the surgical team. A Dutch national program implemented a SSIB in all types of surgeries, including "hygiene discipline" in the OR [49]. Despite the low compliance, the SSI risk was reduced. The multidisciplinary team considered that hygiene discipline, especially in gastrointestinal surgery (i.e., contaminated area), creates a more attentive and accurate work environment and reduces spill of contaminated material. At present, reduction of door movements lacks evidence for its effectiveness.

Bundles that included MBP with oral antibiotics, sterile closure trays and pre-closure gloves changes have significantly greater SSI risk reduction [46]. Few studies have analysed specific incision closure bundles [37-39]. Ghuman et al. did not find any change in SSI rate after implementation of a closure bundle including change in gown and gloves, re-draping, wound lavage and new set of instruments for closure [38]. Limitations of this study are the small sample size and MBP without oral antibiotics. Although literature lacks evidence to support the practice of changing gloves before closure and the use of a specific tray with new instruments, these practices are recommended for CRS [13, 30, 39]. As well, low-quality evidence exists for many other closure preventive measures, such as irrigation, topical antibacterial and antiseptic agents, antibacterial-coated sutures, application of wound sealants, removal of the surgical drape after applying the dressing, antibacterial impregnated dressings and comprehensive postoperative instructions for the patient regarding general hygiene and dressing care. A multicentre randomized trial on rescrubbing before laparotomy closure compared with conventional methods of wound closure did not reduce SSI rate [51]. On the other hand, another study from Japan found that scrubbing the wound with saline and gauze during closure reduced the SSI rates [52]. Although many surgeons irrigate with sterile saline the surgical incision to remove contaminants, there are no guidelines to support a specific type of irrigation fluid, solution additives, delivery method and volume, and it is rarely reflected in most SSIB [39, 50]. Experts have suggested that irrigation with sterile aqueous 0,05% chlorexidine gluconate (CHG) solution is an effective alternative to antibiotic irrigation that lacks efficacy and contributes to bacterial resistance [39, 50]. Coating sutures with triclosan have been used to reduce bacterial attachment to the suture and the formation of a biofilm [39], with a level 1A clinical evidence. The guidelines from the WHO and CDC recommend the use of triclosan-coated sutures as an effective strategy for the prevention of SSI [13, 26, 39]. Ruiz Tovar et al. compared a group of patients with a standard bundle and other group with three additional measures: peritoneal irrigation with gentamicin and clindamycin, fascial closure with triclosan-coated suture and mupirocin ointment application on the skin staples [37]. Statistically significant reductions of incisional (16% vs 2%) and organ-space (4% vs 0%) SSI rates were found with the specific closure bundle.

Unlike most of SSIB focused on elective CRS, Yamamoto et al. developed a successful preventive incisional bundle in patients with colorectal perforation and stoma creation [36]. The rate of SSI was significantly lower after implementation of the bundle (43% vs 20%). The authors included the use of cyanoacrylate tissue adhesive as a wound dressing and an effective barrier against microorganism penetration during stoma creation.

In summary, it can be concluded that preventive SSIB are effective reducing the SSI rate and health costs, especially in CRS. Despite the many different strategies recommended, it is mandatory to reach high levels of compliance and further studies are needed to assess the best cost-effective interventions to achieve better results.

REFERENCES

[1] Fulbrook P, Mooney S. Care bundles in critical care: a practical approach to evidence-based practice. *Nurs Crit Care* 2003; 8 (6): 249-255.

[2] Haraden C. What is a bundle? 2006. *Institute for Healthcare Improvement* (IHI). Available at www.ihi.org/IHI/Topics/Critical-Care/IntensiveCare/ImprovementStories/.

[3] WhatIsaBundle.htm.

[4] Resar R, Griffin FA, Haraden C, Nolan TW. Using care bundles to improve health care quality. IHI Innovation series white paper. Cambridge, Massachusetts: *Institute for Health Improvement* 2012. Avaliable at www.IHI.org.

[5] Berenholtz S, Dorman T, Ngo K, et al. Qualitative review of intensive care unit quality indicators. *J Crit Care* 2002; 17 (1): 1-12.

[6] IHI Shares Achievements of the 5 million Lives Campaign. Press release on October 23, 2008. Cambridge, MA: *Institute for Health*

Care Improvement. Available at http://www.ihi.org/about/news/Documents/IHIPressRelease_IHIShares.
[7] Achievements of5MillionLivesCampaign_Oct08.pdf.
[8] MedQic SCIP Project Information. Available at www.medqic.org/scipn.
[9] Bratzler DW, Houck PM. Antimicrobial prophylaxis for surgery: an advisory statement from the National Surgical Infection Prevention Project. *Am J Surg* 2005; 189: 395-404.
[10] Fry DE. Surgical site infections and the surgical care improvement project (SCIP): evolution of national quality measures. Surg *Infect (Larchmt)* 2008; 9 (6): 579-584.
[11] Khodyakov D, Ridgely MS, Huang C, DeBartolo KO, Sorbero ME, Schneider EC. Project JOINTS: what factors affect bundle adoption in a voluntary quality improvement campaign? *BMJ Qual Saf* 2015; 24 (1): 38-47.
[12] Schwulst SJ, Mazuski JE. Surgical prophylaxis and other complication avoidance care bundles. *Surg Clin N Am* 2012; 92: 285-305.
[13] Marwick C, Davey P. Care bundles: the holy grail of infectious risk management in hospital? *Curr Opin Infect Dis* 2009; 22 (4): 364-369.
[14] Munday GS, Deveaux P, Roberts H, Fry DE, Polk HC. Impact of implementation of the surgical care improvement project and future strategies for improving quality in surgery. *Am J Surg* 2014; 208: 835-840.
[15] Ban KA, Minei JP, Laronga C, Harbrecht BG, Jensen EH, Fry DE, et al. American College of Surgeons and Surgical Infection Society: surgical site infection guidelines, 2016 update. *J Am Coll Surg* 2017; 224 (1): 59-74.
[16] Anderson DJ, Podgorny K, Berrios-Torres SI, Bratzler DW, Dellinger EP, Greene L, et al. Strategies to prevent surgical site infections in acute care hospitals: 2014 update. *Infect Control Hosp Epidemiol* 2014; 35 (6): 605-627.
[17] *Global guidelines on the prevention of surgical site infection.* Geneve: World Health Organization 2016.

[18] European Centre for Disease Prevention and Control. *Surveillance of surgical site infection in Europe 2010-2011*. Available at http://ecdc.europa.eu/en/publications/publicatioons/SSI-in-europe-2010-2011.
[19] Horan TC, Gaynes RP, Martone WJ, Jarvis WR, Emori TG. CDC definitions of nosocomial surgical site infections, 1992: a modification of CDC definitions of surgical wound infection. *Infect Control Hosp Epidemiol* 1992 Oct; 13 (10): 606-8.
[20] Wilson APR, Gibbons C, Reeves BC, Hodgson B, Liu M, Plummer D, et al. Surgical wound infection as a performance indicator: agreement of common definitions of wound infection in 4773 patients. *BMJ* 2004; 25, 329: 720-724.
[21] Solomkin JS, Mazuski J, Blanchard JC, Itani KMF, Ricks P, Dellinger EP, et al. Introduction to the Centers for Disease Control and Prevention and the Healthcare Infection Control Practices Advisory Committee guideline for the prevention of surgical site infections. *Surg Infect* (Larchmt) 2017; 18 (4): 385-393.
[22] Network NHS. *Surgical site infection (SSI) event.* Atlanta, GA: Centers for Disease Control and Prevention, 2019.
[23] Edwards JR, Peterson KD, Mu Y, Banerjee S, Allen-Bridson K, Morrell G, et al. National Healthcare Safety Network (NHSN) report: data summary for 2006 through 2008, issued December 2009. *Am J Infect Control* 2009; 37 (10): 783-805.
[24] Barnes S. Surgical site infection prevention in 2018 and beyond. *AORN J* 2018; 107 (5): 547-550.
[25] Hawn MT, Vick CC, Richman J, Holman W, Deierhoi RJ, Graham LA, et al. Surgical site infection prevention: time to move beyond the surgical care improvement program. *Ann Surg* 2011; 254 (3): 494-499.
[26] National Institute for Health and Clinical Experience (NICE). *Surgical site infection: prevention and treatment of surgical site infection.* NICE, London 2008.
[27] Nguyen N, Yegiyants S, Kaloostian C, Abbas MA, Difronzo LA. The Surgical Care Improvement Project (SCIP) initiative to reduce

infection in elective colorectal surgery: which performance measures affect outcome? *Am Surg* 2008; 74 (10): 1012-1016.

[28] Berríos-Torres SI, Umscheid CA, Bratzler DW, Leas B, Stone EC, Kelz RR, et al. Centers for Disease Control and Prevention Guideline for the Prevention of Surgical Site Infection. *JAMA Surg* 2017; 152 (8): 784-791.

[29] Anderson DJ. Prevention of surgical site infection: beyond SCIP. *AORN J* 2014; 99 (2): 315-319.

[30] Leaper DJ, Tanner J, Kiernan M, Assadian O, Edmiston CE Jr. Surgical site infection: poor compliance with guidelines and care bundles. *International Wound Journal* 2014 (doi: 10.1111/iwj.12243).

[31] Gomez FJ, Fernandez M, Navarro JF. Prevention of surgical site infection: analysis and narrative review of clinical practice guidelines. *Cir Esp* 2017; 95 (9): 490-502.

[32] Cima R, Dankbar E, Lovely J, Pendlimari R, Aronhalt K, Nehring S, et al. Colorectal surgery surgical site infection reduction program: a national surgical quality improvement program-driven multidisciplinary single-institution experience. *J Am Coll Surg* 2013; 216 (1): 23-33.

[33] Lutfiyya W, Parsons D, Breen J. A colorectal "care bundle" to reduce surgical site infections in colorectal surgeries: a single-center experience. *Perm J* 2012; 16 (3): 10-16.

[34] Weiser MR, Gonen M, Usiak S, Pottinger T, Samedy P, Patel D, et al. Effectiveness of a multidisciplinary patient care bundle for reducing surgical site infections. *BJS* 2018; 105: 1680-1687.

[35] Waits SA, Fritze D, Banerjee M, Zhang W, Kubus J, Englesbe MJ, et al. Developing an argument for bundled interventions to reduce surgical site infection in colorectal surgery. *Surgery* 2014; 155 (4): 602-606.

[36] Crolla RMPH, van der Laan L, Veen EJ, Hendriks Y, van Schendel C, Kluytmans J. Reduction of surgical site infections after implementation of a bundle of care. *PLoS ONE* 2012; 7 (9): e44599. Doi:10.1371/journal.pone.0044599.

[37] Keenan JE, Speicher PJ, Nussbaum DP, Adam MA, Miller TE, Mantyh CR, et al. Improving outcomes in colorectal surgery by sequential implementation of multiple standardized care programs. *J Am Coll Surg* 2015; 221 (2): 404-414.

[38] Yamamoto T, Morimoto T, Kita R, Masui H, Kinoshita H, Sakamoto Y, et al. The preventive surgical site infection bundle in patients with colorectal perforation. *BMC Surgery* 2015; 15: 128-133.

[39] Ruiz-Tovar J, Llavero C, Morales V, Gamallo C. Effect of the application of a bundle of three measures (intraperitoneal lavage with antibiotic solution, fascial closure with triclosan-coated sutures and mupirocin ointment application on the skin staples) on the surgical site infection after elective laparoscopic colorectal cancer surgery. *Surgical Endoscopy* 2018 (https://doi.org/10.1007/s00464-018-6069-4).

[40] Ghuman A, Chan T, Karimuddin AA, Brown CJ, Raval MJ, Phang PT. Surgical site infection rates following implementation of a colorectal closure bundle in elective colorectal surgeries. *Dis Colon Rectum* 2015; 58 (11): 1078-1082.

[41] Edmiston CE, Leaper DJ, Barnes S, Jarvis W, Barnden M, Spencer M, et al. An incision closure bundle for colorectal surgery. *AORN Journal* 2018; 107 (5): 552-565.

[42] Tanner J, Kiernan M, Hilliam R, Davey S, Collins E, Wood T, et al. Effectiveness of a care bundle to reduce surgical site infections in patients having open colorectal surgery. *Ann R Coll Surg Engl* 2016; 98: 270-274.

[43] Hoang SC, Klipfel AA, Roth LA, Vress M, Schechter S, Shah N. Colon and rectal surgery surgical site infection reduction bundle: to improve is to change. *Am J Surg* 2019; 217 (1): 40-45.

[44] Lavu H, Klinge MJ, Nowcid LJ, Cohn HE, Grenda DR, Sauter PK, et al. Perioperative surgical care bundle reduces pancreatico duodenectomy wound infections. *J Surg Res* 2012; 174 (2): 215-221.

[45] Hill MV, Holubar SD, Garfield Legare CI, Luurtsema CM, Barth RJ. Perioperative bundle decreases postoperative hepatic surgery infections. *Ann Surg Oncol* 2015; 22 (S3): 1140-1146.

[46] Anthony T, Murray BW, Sum-Ping JT, Lenkovsky F, Vornik VD, Parker BJ, et al. Evaluating an evidence-based bundle for preventing surgical site infection: a randomized trial. *Arch Surg* 2011; 146 (3): 263-269.

[47] Tanner J, Padley W, Assadian O, Leaper D, Kiernan M, Edmiston C. Do surgical care bundles reduce the risk of surgical site infections in patients undergoing colorectal surgery? A systematic review and cohort meta-analysis of 8.515 patients. *Surgery* 2015; 158 (1): 66-77.

[48] Zywot A, Lau CSM, Stephen Fletcher HS, Paul S. Bundles prevent surgical site infections after colorectal surgery: meta-analysis and systematic review. *J Gastrointest Surg* 2017; 21 (11): 1915-1930.

[49] Bull A, Wilson J, Worth LJ, Stuart RL, Gillespie E, Waxman B, et al. A bundle of care to reduce colorectal surgical infections: an Australian experience. *J Hosp Infect* 2011; 78 (4): 297-301.

[50] Holubar SD, Hedrick T, Gupta R, Kellum J, Hamilton M, Gan TJ, et al. American Society for Enhanced Recovery (ASER) and perioperative quality initiative (POQI) joint consensus statement on prevention of postoperative infection within and enhanced recovery pathway for elective colorectal surgery. *Perioper Med* (Lond) 2017; 6 (4). Doi 10.1186/s13741-017-0059-2.

[51] Koek MBG, Hopmans TEM, Soetens LC, Wille JC, Geerlings SE, Vos MC, et al. Adhering to a national surgical care bundle reduces the risk of surgical site infections. *PLoS ONE* 2017; 12 (9): e0184200. https://doi.org/10.1371/journal.pone.0184200; 149 (10): 1045-1052.

[52] Barnes S, Spencer M, Graham D, Johnson HB. Surgical wound irrigation: a call for evidence-based standardization of practice. *Am J Infect Control* 2014; 42 (5): 525-529.

[53] Ortiz H, Armendariz P, Kreisler E, Garcia-Granero E, Espin E, Roig JV, et al. Influence of rescrubbing before laparotomy closure on abdominal wound infection after colorectal cancer surgery: results of a multicenter randomized clinical trial. *Arch Surg* 2012; 147 (7): 614-620.

[54] Goi T, Ueda Y, Nakazawa T, Sawai K, Morikawa M, Yamaguchi A. Measures for preventing wound infections during elective open surgery for colorectal cancer: scrubbing with gauze. *Int Surg* 2014; 99 (1): 35-39.

ABOUT THE EDITORS

Jaime Ruiz-Tovar, MD, PhD
General and Digestive Surgeon
Rey Juan Carlos University Hospital, Madrid, Spain

Professor Jaime Ruiz-Tovar is the Head of the Neurostimulation Unit at Garcilaso Clinic (Madrid, Spain). He is a Bariatric Surgeon at Centro de Excelencia para el Tratamiento de la Obesidad (Valladolid, Spain) and Rey Juan Carlos University Hospital (Madrid, Spain). Dr. Ruiz-Tovar is also a Professor of Surgery, Universidad Alfonso X (Madrid, Spain), and Head of the ERAS-Spain group in Bariatric Surgery

Andrés García Marín, MD, PhD
General and Digestive Surgeon. Hospital Hellín, Albacete, Spain

Dr. Andrés García-Marín is a General and Digestive Surgeon at Hospital de Hellín in Albacete, Spain.

INDEX

A

acute respiratory distress syndrome, 29, 159
additives, 96, 101, 103, 181
adhesion, 126, 128, 143, 144, 155, 157
adhesive properties, 157
adhesives, 98, 156, 159
adults, 23, 79, 144, 149
adverse effects, 19, 49, 75, 109
adverse event, 68, 76, 127, 147
algorithm, 77, 80
allergic reaction, 37, 86, 157
anaphylaxis, 164, 165
anastomotic leakage, 41, 43, 46
antibiotic, v, vii, 36, 41, 42, 43, 44, 45, 46, 47, 48, 49, 50, 51, 52, 53, 68, 74, 103, 105, 106, 107, 109, 115, 117, 119, 120, 121, 122, 123, 124, 125, 130, 136, 138, 142, 154, 159, 164, 165, 166, 167, 168, 177, 181, 186
antibiotic prophylaxis, 47, 50, 51, 52, 53, 68, 74, 117, 142, 177
antimicrobial sutures, 141, 149
antiseptic(s), vi, 2, 36, 39, 55, 56, 57, 59, 60, 63, 81, 86, 96, 97, 101, 103, 107, 108, 114, 116, 119, 120, 126, 141, 143, 144, 153, 154, 155, 156, 158, 164, 166, 167, 168, 181
appendectomy, 115, 117
assessment, 22, 23, 24, 28, 30, 66, 78, 110, 139, 173
atmospheric pressure, 130, 133
avoidance, 66, 143, 155, 183

B

bacteria, 12, 13, 36, 56, 81, 83, 87, 96, 97, 98, 102, 103, 113, 120, 121, 124, 126, 133, 135, 155, 159, 167, 176
bacterial colonies, 121
base, 59, 62, 85, 99, 104, 109, 116, 117, 139, 142, 143, 148, 149, 159, 164, 167, 171, 173, 174, 177, 178, 182, 187
beneficial effect, 71, 85, 145
benefits, 25, 35, 68, 107, 119, 126, 147, 156, 157, 159, 163, 164
bias, 122, 160, 161, 165, 166
biliary tract, 6, 82, 84, 85
bleeding, vii, 50, 70, 72, 134, 154, 159, 167
blood, 66, 67, 69, 72, 75, 76, 78, 80, 87, 99, 104, 120, 133, 134, 173
blood flow, 66, 69, 133

blood transfusion, 173
body composition, 22, 50
body mass index, 10, 50, 82
bowel, 11, 27, 41, 42, 45, 46, 65, 82, 98, 122, 126, 156, 177
bowel obstruction, 27, 98, 126
bundles, vi, vii, 70, 74, 136, 142, 143, 171, 172, 173, 174, 175, 178, 179, 181, 182, 183, 185, 187

C

caesarean section, 162
cancer, 22, 31, 32, 46, 48, 61, 89, 92, 115, 148, 150, 186, 187, 188
carbon dioxide, 28, 157
cardiac surgery, 12, 88, 91, 109, 139, 177
CDC, 3, 5, 14, 30, 60, 92, 142, 147, 149, 173, 175, 181, 184
changing environment, 98
chemical, 2, 37, 38, 57, 101, 126, 159, 167
cholecystectomy, 51, 53, 163
chronic obstructive pulmonary disease, 32, 68
chronic renal failure, 122
classification, 6, 14, 29, 86, 150, 155
clinical trials, 36, 46, 59, 68, 83, 103, 144, 145, 146, 147, 149
closure, 88, 91, 93, 94, 98, 99, 106, 107, 110, 111, 125, 130, 138, 141, 143, 144, 148, 150, 155, 157, 159, 164, 167, 180, 181, 186, 187
clousure, 94
colon, 45, 98, 115, 122, 124, 128, 143, 150
colorectal cancer, 22, 31, 46, 61, 89, 92, 148, 150, 186, 187, 188
colorectal surgery, 5, 7, 14, 41, 42, 45, 46, 52, 68, 74, 90, 122, 124, 127, 142, 144, 146, 148, 149, 150, 161, 162, 172, 176, 177, 178, 179, 185, 186, 187
community, 15, 23

compliance, 26, 150, 172, 174, 175, 178, 180, 182, 185
complications, 7, 17, 21, 24, 28, 46, 48, 55, 56, 61, 68, 70, 71, 76, 78, 79, 81, 94, 95, 127, 130, 131, 136, 137, 142, 148, 149, 172, 173
composition, 22, 50
compounds, 58, 59, 87, 89, 159
consensus, 23, 25, 31, 45, 75, 93, 107, 178, 187
Consensus, 169
contact dermatitis, 164, 165, 166, 167
contamination, 2, 6, 9, 56, 83, 85, 91, 101, 102, 103, 119, 120, 121, 125, 126, 134, 135, 142, 143, 145, 147, 148, 155, 161, 162, 177
controlled trials, 38, 40, 42, 79, 91, 95, 134, 150, 164, 173
controversial, 12, 50, 108, 109, 119, 154
cooling, 78
coronary artery bypass graft, 16
cytokines, 102, 120

D

debridement, 12, 158
decontamination, 101, 156
dehiscence, 135, 146, 147
dermatitis, 164, 165, 166, 167
diabetes, 10, 20, 48, 75, 82, 112, 133, 176
diabetic patients, 66, 74, 75, 112
dissatisfaction, 42
distribution, 49, 123
DOI, 39, 52, 62, 96, 110, 111, 113
drainage, 6, 12, 50, 97, 115, 123, 158, 159, 176
dressings, 89, 110, 131, 133, 137, 153, 154, 155, 156, 157, 158, 159, 160, 161, 162, 163, 164, 168, 181
drugs, viii, 70, 109, 121, 124, 125, 126
duodenum, 49

E

economic problem, 56
emergency, 22, 71, 82, 95, 113, 114, 162, 176
endotracheal intubation, 68
environment, 9, 69, 82, 93, 157, 158, 159, 180
environmental contamination, 155
epidemiology, v, 1, 2, 6, 14, 15, 17, 48, 61, 94, 97, 111, 114, 169, 177
equipment, 72, 100, 177
evidence, viii, 6, 12, 21, 26, 27, 32, 35, 36, 38, 39, 41, 43, 45, 47, 50, 52, 55, 58, 59, 60, 62, 66, 67, 74, 75, 76, 77, 78, 80, 83, 85, 86, 87, 88, 89, 93, 94, 99, 100, 101, 104, 105, 106, 107, 108, 109, 116, 117, 119, 126, 134, 139, 141, 142, 143, 145, 146, 147, 148, 149, 154, 156, 157, 160, 161, 163, 164, 165, 166, 169, 171, 172, 173, 174, 177, 178, 180, 181, 182, 187
evolution, 48, 156, 172, 173, 183
exposure, 37, 69, 83, 101, 106, 134, 154, 155, 156, 160, 161, 163
exudate, 155, 158, 160

F

fascia, 4, 97, 124, 176
fatty acids, 26, 29, 144
fluid, 21, 42, 66, 72, 76, 77, 78, 100, 102, 106, 124, 131, 132, 133, 134, 157, 159, 181
fluid management, 76, 77
Food and Drug Administration, 87, 97
formation, 97, 99, 128, 133, 134, 155, 181
fungal infection, 158

G

gastrointestinal tract, 6
general anaesthesia, 68
general anesthesia, 13, 67, 68
general surgery, 154
glucose, 66, 74, 75, 76, 78, 80, 112, 177
glycosylation, 74
greed, 77
growth, 120, 121, 124, 144, 159
guidelines, 2, 4, 14, 23, 32, 33, 46, 53, 58, 70, 77, 79, 84, 85, 86, 91, 97, 101, 102, 104, 105, 117, 150, 153, 154, 163, 181, 183, 185
guilty, 116

H

haemostasis, 10
hair, 35, 36, 37, 38, 39, 40, 74, 142, 177
hand hygiene, 55, 61, 177
healing, 6, 12, 13, 21, 48, 51, 76, 89, 93, 94, 98, 99, 100, 101, 102, 104, 113, 121, 128, 130, 133, 134, 135, 136, 154, 155, 156, 157, 158, 159, 160, 163, 164, 168
health care, viii, 22, 30, 36, 42, 61, 66, 70, 74, 82, 94, 106, 108, 112, 149, 176, 182
health care costs, 22, 74
hemostasis, vii, 99, 142
heterogeneity, 86, 105, 165, 166
hip replacement, 16, 17
hiperglycemia, 66
homes, 23
hospitalization, 7, 14, 15, 110, 112, 176
host, 67, 97, 142
human, 69, 102, 119, 121, 126
hydrogen peroxide, 101, 158
hygiene, 55, 56, 61, 177, 180, 181
hyperglycaemia, 66, 74, 75
hypothermia, 66, 69, 70, 71, 73, 78, 79
hypothesis, 51, 83, 120, 131

I

ideal, 25, 57, 66, 75, 98, 108, 154, 156, 167
identification, 21, 22, 31
ileus, 41, 43, 44
immune response, 10, 20, 21, 102
immune system, 21, 28, 142
immunosuppression, 48, 51
immunosuppressive therapies, 176
incidence, vii, 1, 2, 6, 7, 20, 22, 26, 36, 37, 48, 57, 59, 70, 81, 84, 88, 95, 110, 115, 117, 125, 129, 130, 137, 141, 142, 143, 144, 149, 164, 175
incision, 4, 5, 20, 37, 50, 59, 60, 66, 67, 85, 86, 87, 88, 89, 90, 91, 93, 94, 97, 107, 108, 122, 127, 129, 130, 131, 132, 134, 137, 138, 142, 148, 167, 177, 181, 186
incision management, 129, 137, 138
induction, 27, 68, 71, 72, 73
inflammation, 6, 100, 120, 134
injury, 28, 33, 99, 114, 158
inoculum, 48, 142
institutions, 172, 177
insulation, 155, 158
insulin, 27, 33, 74, 80
insulin resistance, 74
intensive care unit, 7, 127, 172, 173, 182
International Classification of Diseases, 175
intervention, 21, 22, 23, 24, 51, 67, 72, 95, 124, 129, 136, 142, 172, 175, 176
intra-abdominal abscess, 122
intravenous antibiotics, 44, 109
iodine, 57, 58, 59, 60, 86, 101, 107, 108, 112, 114, 116, 117, 127, 158, 159, 167
irrigation, 69, 73, 93, 94, 95, 97, 100, 101, 102, 103, 104, 105, 106, 107, 108, 109, 110, 111, 113, 114, 115, 116, 117, 119, 120, 121, 122, 124, 125, 126, 130, 181, 187

J

joints, 157

K

kill, 167
knee arthroplasty, 138

L

laboratory studies, 106
laceration, 101, 114
laparoscopic cholecystectomy, 51, 53, 163
laparotomy, 7, 84, 90, 95, 111, 181, 187
latissimus dorsi, 138
lead, 23, 94, 126, 143, 144
leakage, 41, 43, 46, 155
liquid monomer, 159
local anesthesia, 13
love, 56
lymphatic system, 138
lysine, 74

M

majority, 95, 99, 102
malnutrition, 19, 20, 21, 22, 23, 24, 27, 28, 29, 30, 31, 32, 82, 176
management, vii, 12, 53, 76, 77, 79, 80, 89, 94, 98, 100, 101, 104, 110, 113, 114, 120, 129, 137, 138, 142, 156, 173, 175, 183
manipulation, 82, 130, 155, 157, 167
mass, 10, 21, 23, 28, 50, 82
materials, 1, 3, 9, 120, 132, 149
mean arterial pressure, 77
measurement, 71, 161, 173
mechanical bowel preparation, 41, 42, 45, 46, 122, 177

medical, viii, 16, 17, 22, 23, 78, 81, 94, 100, 154, 175
mellitus, 10, 15, 82, 176
meta-analysis, 15, 30, 33, 37, 38, 39, 40, 42, 43, 45, 46, 51, 52, 53, 59, 63, 74, 75, 79, 80, 85, 86, 87, 90, 91, 104, 111, 112, 121, 144, 145, 146, 147, 148, 149, 150, 151, 187
methodology, 103, 145, 172
microbial communities, 97
microbiology, 2, 8, 12, 14, 15, 47, 49
microorganisms, 20, 37, 49, 56, 57, 121, 123, 124, 125
moisture, 87, 157, 158, 159
morbidity, 22, 24, 41, 42, 43, 44, 56, 66, 70, 74, 77, 81, 95, 120, 142
mortality, 8, 9, 14, 22, 24, 41, 42, 43, 44, 56, 74, 80, 81, 95, 112, 120, 121, 123, 142, 172, 176
mortality rate, 8, 41, 95, 121

N

nausea, 79, 164
necrosis, 97, 135
necrotizing fasciitis, 97
negative pressure wound therapy, 129, 137, 138, 139
nerve, 57, 69
neural network, 114
normovolemia, vi, 65, 66, 76, 77, 78
nosocomial pneumonia, 123
nursing home, 23
nutrient, 21, 24, 26, 28
nutrition, 21, 22, 23, 24, 25, 26, 27, 28, 31, 32
nutritional status, 9, 20, 21, 23, 25, 27, 32, 48
nutritional support, 20, 27, 28, 29, 33

O

obesity, 20, 48, 142, 176
obstruction, 27, 98, 126
operations, 6, 84, 116, 120, 136, 149, 150, 180
oral antibiotic, 41, 42, 43, 44, 45, 46, 143, 181
oral antibiotic prophylaxis, 41, 42, 45
oral antibiotics, 43, 44, 46, 181
organ, 4, 5, 48, 97, 130, 147, 176, 178, 180, 182
organs, 1, 3, 4, 11, 69, 142
oxygen, 28, 67, 68, 76, 77, 79, 133, 135, 138, 177
oxygenation, 66, 76, 77, 78, 135, 159

P

pain, 7, 155, 161, 163, 173
partial completion, 174
participants, 36, 83, 145, 161, 162, 163, 164, 165, 166
pathogens, vii, 1, 2, 8, 9, 56, 76, 91, 98, 106, 133
pathway, 32, 45, 56, 187
pectoralis major, 138
performance indicator, 184
perfusion, 66, 77, 78, 135, 139
peripheral vascular disease, 162
peritoneal cavity, 85, 120, 121, 124
peritoneal irrigation, 119, 120, 121, 122, 126, 181
peritoneal lavage, 97, 112, 116, 124, 127, 128
peritonitis, 117, 120, 121, 122, 124, 126, 127, 128, 144
peroxide, 101, 114, 158
phagocytosis, 74
plastic wound protectors, 81, 82
platelet aggregation, 99

population, 3, 16, 23, 57, 80, 96, 103, 112, 138, 167
preoperative bath and shower, 35
preoperative hair removal, 35, 37, 39, 40
prevention, vi, 2, 4, 14, 20, 33, 36, 38, 39, 41, 45, 46, 51, 52, 55, 56, 58, 62, 63, 65, 66, 69, 70, 74, 76, 77, 79, 86, 87, 89, 90, 91, 92, 94, 96, 97, 99, 103, 107, 108, 110, 111, 112, 115, 116, 117, 135, 136, 137, 138, 139, 142, 146, 147, 148, 149, 150, 153, 154, 160, 161, 164, 168, 169, 173, 175, 178, 181, 183, 184, 185, 187
prophylactic, viii, 68, 78, 82, 95, 105, 115, 117, 122, 124, 125, 126, 130, 138, 141, 147, 173
prophylaxis, v, 10, 19, 20, 41, 42, 43, 44, 45, 47, 48, 49, 50, 51, 52, 53, 68, 74, 104, 117, 122, 125, 129, 136, 142, 149, 156, 172, 173, 177, 183
protection, 82, 84, 85, 90, 91, 110, 111, 124, 132, 158
Pseudomonas aeruginosa, 8, 39, 98, 123

Q

quality improvement, 183, 185
quality of life, 22, 24, 30, 56, 61, 129, 142, 148

R

radiotherapy, 22
randomized controlled clinical trials, 46
recommendations, vii, 19, 23, 26, 27, 29, 45, 52, 60, 62, 76, 77, 78, 83, 85, 86, 89, 97, 99, 100, 102, 104, 106, 117, 139, 141, 146, 148, 177
recovery, 27, 31, 36, 42, 45, 46, 70, 72, 73, 172, 187
rectum, 45, 71, 123, 150
regeneration, 93, 104, 116

regression analysis, 75, 145
renal failure, 122
requirements, 21, 28, 157, 176
resection, 14, 46, 82, 97, 98, 127, 150
resistance, 8, 9, 36, 39, 74, 76, 105, 108, 109, 113, 127, 164, 167, 181
respiratory distress syndrome, 29, 159
response, 10, 20, 21, 28, 48, 69, 74, 76, 93, 99, 102, 105, 126, 133
risk factors, 2, 14, 15, 16, 17, 19, 20, 48, 82, 114, 133, 148, 150, 176, 177
risk management, 183
risks, 29, 68, 108, 117, 155, 156, 159, 163, 172

S

scar tissue, 155
scientific knowledge, 174
sensitivity, 27, 165, 166, 176
sepsis, 21, 29, 123, 128, 175
signs, 12, 29, 98, 157
silver, 89, 92, 156, 159, 161, 162, 163, 167
skin, 1, 3, 4, 5, 10, 20, 35, 36, 37, 39, 49, 55, 56, 57, 59, 60, 62, 63, 69, 81, 82, 83, 86, 87, 88, 91, 92, 97, 104, 106, 107, 126, 130, 133, 134, 135, 139, 142, 143, 144, 148, 150, 155, 156, 157, 158, 159, 164, 167, 176, 177, 182, 186
skin antiseptics, 35, 36, 39, 62
solutions, 57, 58, 59, 60, 93, 94, 96, 97, 101, 103, 104, 105, 109, 121, 122, 127, 154
Spain, 1, 7, 8, 15, 35, 41, 47, 55, 65, 81, 119, 129, 141, 143, 153, 171, 189
sponge, 57
standardization, 109, 116, 187
staphylococci, 2, 8
state, 17, 27, 61, 62, 103
sterile, 6, 9, 37, 56, 58, 59, 60, 81, 86, 87, 89, 98, 110, 124, 133, 159, 177, 181
steroids, 158

Index

subcutaneous tissue, 4, 107, 124, 143, 148, 176
supplementation, 26
surgical hand antisepsis, 55, 57, 62
surgical site infection, 1, 2, 3, 4, 10, 14, 15, 16, 19, 20, 21, 30, 31, 33, 35, 36, 39, 40, 41, 42, 46, 47, 48, 52, 53, 55, 56, 62, 65, 66, 70, 71, 76, 77, 78, 79, 80, 81, 82, 89, 90, 91, 92, 93, 94, 95, 99, 108, 109, 110, 111, 112, 115, 116, 117, 129, 130, 137, 139, 141, 148, 149, 150, 151, 153, 154, 163, 166, 169, 172, 175, 176, 183, 184, 185, 186, 187
surgical skin preparation, 55
surgical technique, 21, 48, 81, 123, 134, 176
surgical-site infection, vii, 14, 25, 45, 80, 89, 112, 119, 129, 141, 142, 149, 150
surveillance, 5, 7, 15, 16, 149, 175
suture, 5, 98, 141, 143, 144, 145, 147, 148, 149, 156, 181
synergistic effect, vii, 124

T

target, 28, 66, 75, 76, 77, 78, 80, 142, 159, 177, 180
techniques, 21, 55, 81, 98, 99, 113, 123
technology, 130, 149
temperature, 66, 69, 70, 71, 72, 73, 78, 83
tensile strength, 99
tension, vii, 67, 76
therapy, 26, 31, 32, 36, 42, 51, 66, 76, 77, 80, 127, 129, 131, 132, 137, 138, 139, 176
tissue, 4, 6, 9, 10, 49, 57, 66, 76, 77, 93, 94, 96, 97, 98, 99, 100, 101, 102, 104, 105, 115, 116, 117, 124, 132, 135, 143, 148, 155, 156, 157, 159, 167, 176, 182
topical antibiotics, 103, 105, 108, 116, 125, 153, 154, 160, 163, 164, 165, 166, 167, 168

toxicity, 50, 57, 104, 126
trauma, 6, 10, 76, 98, 105, 137, 155, 157, 158
treatment, 6, 7, 12, 13, 21, 66, 75, 79, 81, 88, 91, 93, 95, 110, 112, 121, 125, 127, 128, 130, 138, 164, 167, 172, 184
trial, 33, 38, 40, 52, 53, 60, 85, 88, 90, 91, 92, 95, 107, 110, 111, 115, 116, 117, 122, 128, 148, 149, 165, 178, 181, 187
triclosan-coated sutures, 141, 144, 145, 146, 147, 148, 149, 150, 181, 186

U

undernutrition, 22, 23, 31
urinary bladder, 71
urinary tract, 6, 20
urinary tract infection, 20

V

vacuum, 131, 159
vancomycin, 49, 50, 109, 159
variables, 9, 101, 124
variations, 96, 103
vascular surgery, 5, 92, 137
vascularization, 156
vasoconstriction, 69, 70
ventilation, 10, 20
viruses, 57, 167

W

water, 57, 58, 59, 101, 155, 158, 160, 164
weight loss, 21, 24
work environment, 180
World Health Organization, 4, 14, 20, 30, 33, 38, 62, 79, 91, 104, 106, 107, 115, 136, 146, 177, 183
wound dehiscence, 135, 146, 147

wound healing, 6, 21, 94, 99, 100, 101, 104, 121, 128, 135, 136, 156, 159
wound infection, 3, 13, 14, 15, 30, 37, 62, 76, 80, 81, 82, 90, 91, 97, 98, 101, 113, 114, 115, 116, 117, 121, 123, 124, 125, 137, 138, 149, 157, 160, 167, 176, 184, 186, 187, 188
wound irrigation, 93, 94, 95, 100, 101, 102, 103, 105, 106, 107, 108, 109, 111, 114, 116, 117, 130, 187
wound management, 94, 98, 100, 101, 104, 110
wounds, 2, 6, 82, 94, 97, 98, 99, 100, 102, 104, 105, 106, 107, 113, 116, 130, 133, 135, 153, 155, 156, 157, 158, 159, 160, 161, 162, 163, 164, 167, 168, 170

Z

zinc, 165

Related Nova Publications

PROPHYLAXIS IN BARIATRIC SURGERY

EDITOR: Jaime Ruiz-Tovar, M.D., Ph.D.

SERIES: Surgery – Procedures, Complications, and Results

BOOK DESCRIPTION: The aim of this book is to revise the actual evidence of the most important prophylactic measures that a morbidly obese patient must undergo.

SOFTCOVER ISBN: 978-1-53613-435-3
RETAIL PRICE: $95

GASTRIC BYPASS SURGERY: PROCEDURES, BENEFITS AND HEALTH RISKS

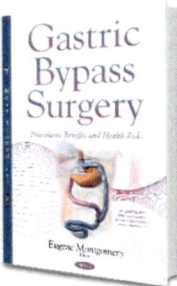

EDITOR: Eugene Montgomery

SERIES: Surgery – Procedures, Complications, and Results

BOOK DESCRIPTION: Obesity is a multifactorial global epidemic with associated risk factors for an array of vascular, metabolic, psychological and economical consequences. Bariatric surgery has revealed a significant link between gastrointestinal metabolism and obesity that extends to resolution of many metabolic diseases including type 2 diabetes and cardiovascular disease risk.

SOFTCOVER ISBN: 978-1-63485-412-2
RETAIL PRICE: $95

To see complete list of Nova publications, please visit our website at www.novapublishers.com